FIND OUT WHAT TURNS HIM ON . . .

Fire

Aries: The more you ignore him, the hotter he'll get. So go ahead and tease him into submission.

Air

Gemini: Flirting is second nature to Gemini, so rope him in with your sheer wit and sexy banter.

Earth

Virgo: Virgo loves dating up and image is very important to him. If you've got a pedigree or an impressive career, make sure to let him know.

Water

Pisces: He is a pretty boy who can make you fall in love with him at first sight. Seduce him by wearing your heart on your sleeve.

Acclaim for
THE CELESTIAL SEXPOT'S HANDBOOK

W9-BUO-567

more . . .

"Kiki knows exactly how you'll be getting lucky."

—*Scarlet* (UK)

"Sexy, funny, and stunningly accurate! Kiki is a shining star . . . This cosmic guide is laugh-out-loud! Kiki truly knows the ins and outs of the zodiac's men!"

—Tali Edut, cofounder of Astrostyle.com and coauthor of *Astrostyle: Star-studded Advice for Love, Life and Looking Good*

"Kiki is *the* go-to-girl for spot-on descriptions of what makes your lover tick. Once you've read this book, seduction will never be the same . . . Read it now and your bed will never be empty again."

—Stefanie Iris Weiss, coauthor of *Surviving Saturn's Return: Overcoming The Most Tumultuous Time of Your Life* and astrologer of British *Elle*

"This book has more helpful ideas about love and lust than a sex counselors' convention. Armed with wit and wisdom, Kiki clears twelve new paths on the road to a relationship."

—Jeff Jawer, cofounder of StarIQ.com and coauthor of *Your Astrology Guide*

"Finally, an astrology book that gives us what we really want, the down-and-dirty details on how to bed, bag or, if necessary even break with a guy based on his sign. You'll thank your lucky stars for this thorough, foolproof guide! Read it and you'll have his stars aligned with yours in no time flat!"

—Jaime Harkin, *In Touch Weekly*

THE
CELESTIAL
SEXPOT'S
HANDBOOK

ASTROLOGICAL TIPS FOR SATISFYING SEDUCTION AND ULTIMATE LOVE

KIKI T.

WARNER BOOKS

NEW YORK   BOSTON

To: Simon Le Bon,
the man who started it all, giving me
my first case of the astral panty sweats . . .
and to all the men I've loved before,
who traveled In and out my door,
I'm glad they came along . . .

Warner Books
Hachette Book Group USA
1271 Avenue of the Americas
New York, NY 10020
Visit our Web site at www.HachetteBookGroupUSA.com

Warner Books and the "W" logo are trademarks of Time Warner Inc.
or an affiliated company. Used under license by Hachette Book
Group, USA, which is not affiliated with Time Warner Inc.

Printed in the United States of America

First Edition: January 2007
10 9 8 7 6 5 4 3 2 1

Library of Congress Cataloging-in-Publication Data
Tom, Karen.
The celestial sexpot's handbook : astrological tips for satisfying seduction and ultimate love
/ Kiki T. — 1st ed.
p.   cm.
Summary: "A sex and astrology guide in one — provides the tools to help readers find the
man of their dreams and the ultimate satisfaction with him." — Provided by the publisher.
ISBN-13: 978-0-446-69695-1
ISBN-10: 0-446-69695-1
1. Astrology and sex.   2. Love — Miscellanea.   I. Title.
BF1729.S4T66   2007
133.5'864677 — dc22   2006010678

Book design by JoAnne Metsch

Acknowledgments

A special thanks to . . .

Mary Tahan, my double Aries agent extraordinaire with the killer instincts to be the first to fall in love with this book.

Andie Avila, my Gemini editor, thanks especially for diplomatically dealing with all my double Scorpio obsessing and tirelessly quelling all my issues.

My editors at *Jane*, Tina Chadha and Stephanie Trong.

My editors at *Playgirl*, Jill Sieracki and Michelle Zipp—for making me a Playgirl.

Tali Edut, fellow astrologist and Scorpio moon. Thanks for your endless Sagittarian optimism and your four-planets-in-Scorpio-persistent support through everything, this book and beyond! You seriously amaze me!

Mina Takata. Thanks for your eternal belief in me and always knowing what to say and when to say it. Plus, you're too much fun and as cute as a button—I love you like crazy!

Christine Sauertieg. You define what friendship means to me, completely! There's hardly a bad time with you—and that includes over half my life of knowing you!

John Sampson. I get happy just thinking about you—especially your totally evil sense of humor, hee hee. I love our friendship and thankfully it's forever!

Yusuf Gatewood. Even without our contract, I'd love you endlessly. Now get me to Morocco!

Monica Lawrence, aka Moniq'wah. I better thank you, you have too much blackmail on me not to. lol. xoxo!

Meena Hwang, aka Muh. Long live the brain cell and our "Dandi" lives!

Jocelyn Charvet. What would I do without all your insight?

Michael Agard. Thanks for your genius and bailing me out of all my technical messes!

Gina, Bora, and Sophie. For all your positive energy! Love you all to bits!

Brad Heckman, Arion SoRelle (aka Lala), Lois Sakany, Julie Guarino, and Jay Venute—kisses and love to you all for your fabulously supportive friendships.

. . . and always and forever, love to the Bauddha, without you, life would have been a disaster!

Contents

Introduction

The only question you ever need to ask to get what you want is: "When's your birthday?"

— KIKI

Dial 4-1-1 . . . Hello, Miss Kiki on the line . . .

Congratulations, you've just made the smartest purchase of your life. After all, what other item can help you get *everything* you want, from *whomever* you want? Certainly nothing legal I can think of . . . Yes, within these pages are delectable tidbits of information that'll allow you to enter into a hedonistic paradise where you're the boss and everyone else is your willing minion. Just by finding out one's birthday, you can unlock anyone's star-crossed secrets, allowing you to emotionally judo-flip him to his back, knees, or wherever you want— everything to woo, coo, do, and even shoo him, if you want.

While this may sound too good to be true, it's not!

"Ooh, tell me more . . ."

Chances are you're already an avid astrology buff—after all, why else would you pick this book up. If not, you're probably a desperate cynic who has reached depraved levels of lust/love and is praying this book will help in your salvation. Either way, you bought this book because you want something and will stop at nothing to get it. Good for you—because that's why astrology was discovered in the first place.

To desire is human nature, and since the inception of civilization we've been looking to the stars to help gain control over this mess called life. After all, wouldn't it be absurd to think the universe beyond us didn't influence us in any way? Our predecessors obviously knew planetary forces shaped us and our destinies—and evidence of the use of horoscopes dates back to 4200 BC. In fact, all ancient cultures— from the Babylonians, Greeks, Chinese, Hindus, and Romans— discovered an astrological system with twelve symbols of similar meaning and all systems were created independently of one another.

Of course, in our cynical age I'm always getting those snide people telling me astrology is bullshit. Sure, there's no hard evidence of why it works, but it's how it works that makes it so riveting—much like gravity, time, or any other invisible concept. For those people who scoff at astrology, they can think what they sadly want. I've had it work for me and seen it work for others and the proof is in the pudding. And hey, can zillions of people throughout history be nuts?

So, while I can babble facts and theories for astrology's validity, the only real way to prove it is to challenge any naysayers to the ole "seeing is believing" method. If you're a doubter, just try these tips and watch yourself get what you desire; then you'll know the power of this ancient science and embrace it as your own. After all, who doesn't want it his or her way? (And for those of you who never want to give in, you can always use this book to manipulate those astral cultists.)

However, because I'm a generous individual, I'll throw in a few particulars and a shot of peer pressure just because they're fun facts to know. Take note:

♡ Suicide rates go up and hospitals report more hemorrhaging in surgery on full moons.

♡ Typically, computers break down, communication is disrupted, negotiations are slowed, and/or people from the past tend

to return while Mercury (planet of communication) is retrograde (when a planet is seemingly moving backward).

♋ When sunspots flare up, the stock market plummets or rises
just as dramatically.

♋ Smart people use astrology. Followers have included Pythago-
ras, Christopher Columbus, Sir Isaac Newton, Charles de
Gaulle, Winston Churchill, Carl Jung, T.S. Eliot, and J.P. Mor-
gan, who brilliantly stated, "Millionaires don't use astrology;
billionaires do."

So, do I really live by this stuff?

You better believe it! I'm an astral addict—however, I'm no starlit
junkie. While I look to see where the planets are, I don't live every
minute dictated by charts. I'm a firm believer in fate and free will,
and I think that everyone is born with a special mission and abilities
and that astrology can serve as a reference for getting in touch with
that potential—via a birth chart. It's free will that then says how far
you want to take that potential.

I think of astrology the same way I think of weather, but instead of
climates, it's about energy. By knowing where the planets are and
how they're interacting, I can gauge which events would be more
auspicious or less favorable during certain periods. However, I
know I need to put out the effort to work with that energy. Astrology
doesn't make things happen, it just helps me—or you—make things
happen. For example, with weather, if you know it's going to rain,
you don't plan a picnic. Astrology works in the same way. If there're
bad aspects, you plan around them. If there're good ones, you plan
for them. When a planet is in retrograde, expect trouble in the area
that planet rules. If Venus, the planet of love and art, is retrograde,
chances are beauty treatments won't go as smoothly as they could.
Projects started during a new moon tend to have a higher success

rate. If the sun is in Leo, a fire sign, and you're an Aries, another fire sign, expect a creative boost. Once you learn the basic gist of each sign and what the placements of planets mean, the task of using astrology becomes very easy and soon enough, second nature.

How did I wind up this way?

Like any self-respecting double-Scorpio, I was lured in because of an obsession. At the age of eleven I was in dire love with Simon Le Bon of Duran Duran. It was the height of my cruel adolescence, and my only escape was through fantasies of one day uniting with Simon, aka my soul mate—and a Scorpio like me. Astrology confirmed our compatibility; therefore, I became an instant full-fledged believer. The first astrology book I bought: Judith Bennett's *Sex Signs*.

Years later, I learned the finer points of astrology, got off the Simon Le Bon obsession, and realized how potent this starry maze of manipulation was. How I wound up writing about astrology was unexpected, though. Just out of college, having majored in creative writing, someone suggested I pitch an astrology column—as I was always asking people's signs. I took that advice (of course, from an Aries, the ideas people), and my writing career began. The first column I created was for a gay and lesbian publication entitled, "The Celestial Bitch and Butch Report"—with two predictions, each based on your inner bitch or butch. Then, my expertise was focused on the teen scene for several years, until I owned up to what I do best— being smutty. In 2002, I landed my column in *Playgirl*. It was exactly two weeks after a lunar eclipse in my natal first house (the first house represents one's identity), which is a major indicator of change. In January 2003, *Astral Vibrations* debuted and my career as the one and only astrosexologist began.

In 2004, my astro adventures continued when I became the astrologer for *Jane*. This happened one month post a lunar eclipse in the first house of my solar chart (another change in my identity) and on the day of a Venus eclipse (in my second house, the house of money!). But enough about me and about this book . . .

So, okay, here's your crash course to absolute fascism . . .

Sure, while some may think it's a bit nasty to put a book out on how to play people to your liking, we're talking about love in the twenty-first century and we all have to do what we have to do. So, here are my wicked little Scorpio secrets and how to put that knowledge to work for you, at maximum capacity.

As you'll see, each sign/chapter is cut up into four major sections. All of it is devised to smoothly guide you along the general phases of a relationship. Starting at *Bare Basics*, you'll learn how to spot each sign and their methods of seduction, ways to seduce them back, and why you'd want them in the first place. Once you get past that initial phase of the mating ritual, take things to the next level by *Making Him Come to the Palm of Your Hand*. There, you can load up on all the astral dating pointers you'll need to pique his interest and more—everything, including fashion tips, dining ideas, cinematic selections, dating activities, conversational icebreakers, mood music, and gift ideas.

Then, when you're ready to go, blow his mind behind closed doors with star-studded methods on heating him up, including role-playing ideas. After all that, you should know exactly where his emotions lie. However, if you do question his loyalty, get your answer at "Taking the Bait." If he has indeed bitten, then hold tight, because as most of you know, gaining the affections of your man is only half the story. The other half is to know what makes him tick and how to deal. Enter *Astral Autopsy*, where you get to look into the celestial cadaver and see his emotions dissected for your viewing pleasure. Learn how he processes fear, anger, sadness, trust, and motivation— and better yet, how you can cause and quell them at will, too.

If, even after all these libidinous adventures, you discover you're not fully satisfied with your find, no worries. That's what *Destination: Dumpsville* is there for. After all, with love, satisfaction is never guaranteed. So, read the fine print and get the clues to know if you're going to be dumped first and if he hates you, or ways you can effectively beat him to the punch. And because no one likes to go home a sore loser, all chapters wrap up with a positive lesson each sign leaves behind—no matter how miserable the demise. Although, hopefully most of you won't need this section, as you'll have detoured into the happily-ever-after path instead.

Now the advanced stuff . . . Yes, there's more—don't worry; it's worth it . . .

Okay, while everyone knows about their sun sign, that's really only the tip of the astrological iceberg. Along with your sun sign, a birth chart also includes many facets—such as rising sign and moon sign (the two most important aspects in a chart after the sun), and then there are the planets—all of which represent different areas of your personality. The sun rules the basic personality; the rising dictates the social persona, the moon deals with the emotions, Mercury is communication, Venus is pleasure, Mars is drive, Jupiter is optimism, Saturn is discipline, Uranus is innovation, Neptune is idealism, and Pluto is transformation.

During one's birth, the planets' positions in relation to where and when the blessed event occurred bring a welcome wagon of personality influences to that individual. By knowing someone's planetary positions, you can find out what celestial themes make up that special someone's personality, making it easy for you to open the doorway into his psyche. Of course, this doesn't have to be so involved. For those who want straightforward manipulation, go with your intended's sun-sign information. For more intense scrutiny, look up his complete chart on one of the slew of websites (www. astrology3d.com, www.astro.com, www.alabe.com/freechart/) that offer free charts. Then, go for the kill. If Cancer man has four planets in Gemini, read both Cancer and Gemini to get maximum power over him. If his Venus is in Scorpio, flip to Scorpio to find out what tickles his fancy, as far as tastes go. If his Mars is in Virgo, read Virgo to see what motivates him. If his moon is in Taurus, read up on what makes Taurians neurotic and have your fun. It's all about recognizing what astrological influences make up a person and how to use astro intelligence to nail your man.

Of course, if you have to force someone to be with you, then you need more than astrology to help you. This book is to be used only in the promotion of love and happiness, which should be the goal for anyone's life. This book isn't for chasing after a man who repeatedly blows you off or is up in everyone else's ass, because with a loser like that, neither these suggestions nor anything else will ever get him to come around—and you shouldn't want that man to come around anyway.

If you do find yourself in that predicament, it would be better if you read up on your own sign to see what makes you happy. Remember, love is not about controlling others to just get what you need, but what you feel is best for all involved. Sure, in ensuring that happiness, sometimes it requires some manipulation, but if he submits and wants to see you happy, then you know you have someone worth exploring. If he never gives into your needs and there's more misery than merriment, take a hint. Either way, the art of love is a nasty little bitch and sometimes you have to do whatever it takes to get you through. As they say, "All is fair in love and war," and as I'll tell you, "If these tips don't make you more fuckable, I don't know what will!"

Love, Love, Love,
Kiki

Master Manipulation Map

To maximize the celestial secrets found in these pages, go to the Internet and chart out your beloved's astro info and fill in the blanks with his appropriate zodiac sign. Then utilize the following sections to get the most out of your man! For example, if your Honey is a Mars in Leo, flip to Leo and read what gets him angry. Or if he has a Cancer moon, but is a Pisces, look at both signs' seduction methods to turn him on.

While all the planets are essential in knowing the ins and outs of a person's character, with relationships the main categories to be concerned with will be the sun, ascendant, moon, Mercury, Venus, and Mars. Note there could be several sections that can help you bait your traps, so read up on all and get that many more creative ways to nail your man!

Name: _____

Date of Birth: _____

Time of Birth: _____

Place of Birth: _____

Modus Operandi

All Categories   **Sun** (Basic Self) _____

All Categories   **Ascendant** (Social Self) _____
Esp. Key Features

Seducing Him   **Moon**
                    (How He Feels About Love) _____

Loving Him

Taking the Bait

Fear

Sadness

Trust

Celestial Voodoo

Beating Him to the Punch

. . . And Other Signs He Hates You

Kick, Drop, and Kill

Conversation   **Mercury**
                    (Communication Style) _____

Movies

Role-Playing

Trust

Motivation

Beating Him to the Punch

Seducing Him   **Venus**
                    (What Turns Him On) _____

Loving Him

Eye Candy

Food

Movies

Dating Ideas

Music

WANTED: ARIES

BORN: MARCH 21–APRIL 19

Fast-talking narcissist with a penchant for playing devil's advocate. Favorite word: "me." Does not register the word, "No," or much of what anyone else has to say.

BARE BASICS

How to Spot Him

Feeling hot? If so, get ready to have all your senses assaulted by Aries, the aggressive and unapologetic force with a throbbing passion that never ceases. Built with a super-sonar radar, he has an uncanny ability to track down any emission of heat and be on your ass accordingly. Obnoxious, obviously. Captivating, quite overwhelmingly, but as much as you might want to tear yourself away from his seemingly overbearing and arrogant ways, you'll find it isn't quite so easy to escape his in-your-face cocky charisma. Although you'll hate to admit it, he'll pique a twisted curiosity and you'll stay. Besides, you sense that you can run, but unfortunately you can't hide—as this is Aries' way: conquer at any cost.

As you guessed, there's no ignoring this man when he wants your attention. If you try, you're just asking him to turn up his volume. Aries has an infinite number of tricks up his sleeves, and he's willing to pull out every last one of them just to impress you, even if it's just for a second. In fact, the more you resist the more he'll insist, as he thrives on a good challenge. Plus, he's protected by his delusion of invincibility and an ego built like a tank that'll crush rejection. Only if he gets bored will he ease up, but typically, he'll lay on the flattery so thick that you'll eat up his fool-for-love routine. Then, once you start melting in his hands, the adventure begins—the Aries 0–190 mph ride to destination unknown.

Yes, expect the unexpected. Filled with a boundless enthusiasm and a spontaneous spirit, Aries is as unpredictable as they come. Where there's danger, there's Aries, and the more extreme the better. Nothing is too big for him, even his own bark. In love, he's just as bold, as he strives for a love to end all loves each time he enters. Aries isn't the guy to hold back on anything, least of all his feelings, and when smitten will do everything in his power to make sure you're given nothing less than five-star treatment that'll have you thinking the sun rises and sets on you.

Possessing a legendary chivalry, Aries custom-fits himself to his lover's ideal. Being able to juggle many modes, he can be the gentleman of your dreams one minute, your superhero the next, and your fabulous lover-man all the while. Consumed with a desire to be the best, for love, he works his tail off to keep your mind and body inspired beyond your standards. All you'll need to do is saddle up your courage and reserves of energy and be ready to roll with his quicksilver style of love. You know it: An Aries offer is one that rarely a horny person can refuse.

Key Features:

- ♡ A compact/stout build, usually with overly large biceps and short legs/long torso
- ♡ Well-defined facial features and a mop of thick hair
- ♡ Flashy clothes in color or cost—not necessarily stylish either, but bold for sure
- ♡ Wears flashy jewelry and/or too much cologne

♡ Aggressive and combative nature
♡ Loud manner of speaking
♡ Parties to excess in expense and intake

Seducing Him into Your Boudoir

You don't have to burn a lot of calories to bag an Aries. He's so into being the "guy" that all you need to do is sit there, look pretty, and periodically play hard to get until he's on the brink of busting a nut. He gets excited at the thought of conquests, and having to earn it brings out his best. Hell, the more you ignore him, the hotter he'll get. So, go ahead and tease him into your submission. Arouse his senses and raise the stakes; show you're cocky too and play him at his game. Be wild and adventurous. The more insane and fearless you are, the more irresistible you'll be.

By making him see you as an equal and better, he'll gain respect for you. This will give you leverage, as Aries is a self-absorbed Casanova who assumes most people are dying to get with him. Shock him with your self-control and force him to some humility, to approach you on a human level rather than his typical smug form of seduction. The more of a challenge you are, the more you'll see what kind of man he really is. Plus, it'll make him engorged with desire and focus on the sex beyond a physical sense. In seeing you as more than just a plug for his penis it forces him to up the ante on his performance. To Aries, anything hard to get is prestigious, and he's all about being judged on showmanship, especially from someone he reveres.

One warning, though, timing is everything with Aries. Just like spaghetti, there's a small window where he's perfectly al dente. A few seconds after, it's a drippy noodle. He's impatient and wants to feed into the instant gratification of passion—so don't keep the heat on too long. Read him well and give him the go at just the precise moment. Then, bon appétit!

Loving Him in the Boudoir

Aries is passionate and aggressive, and he loves catching people off guard. He lives for spontaneity, but under his terms. He doesn't like to be pinned down, especially in sex and love. His style is hot and heady 24-7, which means you'll get the workout of a lifetime. Living and loving at a furious pace, expect Aries to give you the most bang for your fuck. Be ready to be wrestled with, tossed around, and twisted into positions you never thought possible. Do the same with him, as he loves primal sex.

His one downfall, though, is longevity. While Aries can give you lots of variety and excitement, it'll be on the installment plan. Rather than one long erotic tale that just pushes you inch by inch into an ecstasy so deep you'll think you've popped blood vessels, Aries is a spin cycle: quick and fast, but always ready for the next load. However, even if he's not Mr. Snap and Pop, he won't slag with his sexual program. Being the ruler of the head, the symbol gets played out rather nicely in the boudoir. He can give it and get it eternally, giving your jaws a workout like you couldn't believe.

For the long term, though, know his first impressions are his best. So, if he didn't break out the big guns ASAP, don't bother wasting anymore time waiting for the main event. He's a "take it or leave it" guy. Once he makes his mark, you'll know where his talents lie — which makes it very easy to choose where to go from there. If one memorable night is what you're looking for, you'll have gotten the gold. However, if you dig the goods, then his stout fatty will be sure to please you again — as once he's been somewhere, he likes going back to make sure he's covered all the ground. Just give him a few minutes and get his encore.

MAKING HIM COME TO THE
PALM OF YOUR HAND

Eye Candy

He's vain and in love with himself; adorning himself in the finest vestments is just another excuse to spend time in front of the mirror. Yes, Aries is loud and proud. Take a cue from his power color red and think red carpet—as he thinks he's walking one everywhere he goes. To keep up with Mr. Showbiz, know you're going to have to play the yin to his fashion yang and put together a look that's bright, bold, and brash. There's nothing too flamboyant for Aries, just as long as the glare from your shine isn't outdoing him, then you're good to go.

Stylin' Seduction:

- ♡ Red, his signature color. It'll remind him of victory, courage, and blood—three things he adores.
- ♡ Classic tailored clothes, such as power suits. Looking like you mean business means being able to hold your sexuality with authority.
- ♡ Short hemlines, skintight clothing, or anything overtly sexual. Modesty isn't in his vocabulary.
- ♡ Animal prints. It shows confidence—and the bolder, the better.
- ♡ Trendy and expensive labels. Extra points if you're in the most underground designer duds. He loves being ahead of the trends.
- ♡ Leather. It's got a classic sex vibe to it that can never go wrong with Aries. Plus, leather's association with rebellion makes Aries unable to resist anyone adorned in it.
- ♡ Big hair. All the better if it's the look of just-fucked hair, which is a sexy style he can't deny.

Tasty Treats

Food

Aries are indulgent about everything, and food is just another thing for him to go overboard on. He likes his dining experiences to be big and dramatic and the foods to be rich, intense, decadent, and spicy. However, the deal is he isn't generally a master gourmet; he's more about being seen at the latest places, schmoozing up to anyone he can and paying exorbitant amounts for those bragging rights. That's right, what tastes good to him isn't so much about the spices, but the prices. It's a fact that he won't readily care to admit to, as it's a truth that's hard to swallow.

Erotic Eats:

♡ Any restaurant that's just opened. He loves being the first among his friends to try anything.

♡ Restaurants with expensive prices, a dress code, valet parking, and/or a reputation for top-notch service. A service staff that kisses ass is as good as a fancy dinner in the eyes of Aries!

♡ Any super trendy cuisine or locale. The hipper and more exclusive, the better.

♡ Places that serve exotic meats. For example, a Japanese restaurant that serves blowfish. Aries love to dance with danger!

♡ Spicy foods. He loves to prove his ability to take heat.

♡ BBQ. It can be any kind. As a fire sign, he loves anything cooked with it. However, Korean would be especially great, as he can play with fire (and the food is spicy!).

♡ Brazilian rotisserie restaurants (aka Churrascarias). Snap your fingers, they come, they serve. The power alone will make him salivate. (This is carnivore option only.)

Movies

Aries loves action! He lives for it and won't have the patience for anything less than fast or faster. To get him to sit still for at least ninety minutes will require cinema that's overwhelming, sucking him into a more fantastical slice of life than he can imagine. He wants inspiration—inspiration to live, love, and fight stronger. Sure, that may be asking a lot, but that's him: optimistically demanding. To ensure this kind of experience, he'll opt for cinema that has guts, gore, and glory. Think action-packed adventures, military epics to jam-packed special effects stimuli.

Cinematic Foreplay:

- ♡ Spy/espionage films. He loves anything that deals with conspiracy.
- ♡ War movies. He's the sign of war.
- ♡ Gun-toting male machismo movies, like classic De Niro movies or Tarantino-type films. Violence turns him on. This can also include martial art flicks. Fighting is an Aries thing.
- ♡ New films that've had any hype. He loves to be the first to see anything and offer his opinions as if they're fact. And the more controversial the matter in which to form his opinions, the better.
- ♡ Biographies, particularly on famous leaders. Documentary or fictionalized accounts are fine. He'll think he can relate to them.
- ♡ Melodrama. Anything over the top and he's in.
- ♡ Musicals. He has a soft side, too, and will love the flamboyance of a good song-and-dance number.

Dating Ideas

Aries is a show-off, with tons of energy to burn. He's a high-octane man who flitters on the edge: anything scary, sign him up. He thrives with physical and competitive challenges, as he's typically gifted with an athletic ability and a strategic mind. Take him on wild adventures he's never experienced and he'll worship the ground you walk on. Not only will he love trying something new, he'll love having more to boast about and be able to play critic to others who attempt to follow in his footsteps. Any place where he can take a hit of adrenaline and amp his spirit full of endorphins is where you'll get Aries at his finest.

Playful Planning:

♡ Paintball, laser tag, or any other interactive, competitive, and combative sport. Opposition brings out his true nature.

♡ An extreme sport involving speed. He loves natural rushes.

♡ A shooting range. He's got a thing about firearms.

♡ Off-road adventures. Anything rough is hot to Aries.

♡ Amusement parks with elaborate roller coasters. Again, the adrenaline rush of being shaken up at top speed will give him a thrill.

♡ Shopping. He'll get off on showing off his buying power. If you can take him to a flea market or an auction, even better— negotiating is one of his favorite pastimes.

♡ A protest. Nothing says excitement to Aries more than rebellion.

Sound Seduction

Conversation

Engaging in a conversation with Aries is easy, if you don't mind listening to him talk about himself. Me, me, me is a theme he never gets tired of—but being that he's so charismatic, he can get away with it (at least early on). Therefore, prepare yourself to get more than a handful of information that goes from trivial to personal all in the span of one breath. Not to say you aren't important, you just need to claim your stake. How? By shocking the crap out of him, offering up insane confessional stories of daring adventures or issues that really make him question his morality and can fuel heated discussions. Get him to stop starting all his sentences with an "I." You may wonder if his self-absorption isn't really just a defense mechanism. Oh, the things we wish really could be true.

Icebreakers:

♡ Ask him about what he fears. Get to know what really makes him tick.

♡ Ask him what's the most evil thing he's ever done to anyone. He may water down the truth, but what he'll fess up to is good insight into his ego.

♡ Find out who he hates the most now and why. He's aggressive and passionate; learn how off his rocker he is when you discover who his enemies are.

♡ Raise questions involving money and indulgence; they never fail. Ask how much he spent on his clothes. He'll be more than happy to brag about his clothes and what he spent.

♡ Ask how he thinks other people see him and how he wants to be seen. You can figure out how disillusioned he is from his answers, as most tend to be clueless to their faults.

♡ Play the, "If you were the leader of the world" game. Ask him what he'd change and things he would do. He loves pretending he rules the universe.

♡ Ask what would he do if someone gave him a million tax-free dollars and he had a week to spend it? All Aries are extravagant; find where his true loves lie.

Music

Aries thinks himself a trendsetter, the guy in the know before everyone else. With music, he'll consider himself an expert, giving his mark of excellence as if he's some sort of aficionado. On his turntables:

sultry mood music that hits the chords of primal emotion. He loves anything new, trendy (as in too cool for school, not Top 40 trendy), loud and/or music that overwhelms you into being physical. It's all about being hip or at least seeming it, so be the DJ with the exclusive tracks.

Mood Makers:

- ♡ Underground DJs. Anything deemed hip appeals to his senses.
- ♡ Metal: heavy, speed, and death. He loves anything aggressive.
- ♡ Dance music/disco. He's a physical guy and loves any type of music that he can move to.
- ♡ Indie rock. The newer and more obscure, the better.
- ♡ Rap and hip-hop. Music with a strong beat sets him in the mood.
- ♡ Over-the-top vocalist he can sing along to. Opera would work also. It's all about the drama with this one.
- ♡ Dub, ambient, techno. If it's left of mainstream, go for it. He's into everything found there.

Gifts

Paying the piper is essential to keeping Aries happy. He wants to be showered with love and the more expensive your displays, the better. Extravagance works on him; it shows you think no sacrifice is too big for him. Not to say his love has a price tag, because it doesn't always. It's just that he does tend to get judgmental in this department, a fact he can't hide. As for what you should blow the bank on, think luxury items, rare one-of-a-kind collectibles or anything that can appreciate with value—as he'll wish your love with him will. Corny yes, but so is he.

Boxed Treats:

- ♡ Jewelry. If it's engraved with a personal message, even better. Anything that bears his name on it works, as he's territorial.
- ♡ Clothes. He's a fashion victim through and through. Just don't forget: labels please.
- ♡ Spa treatments. Who is he to say no to being pampered?
- ♡ Stuff for his car. The flashier the better. He lives to travel in style.
- ♡ Trips. Think extravagant and romantic.
- ♡ Sporting equipment. He's a jock-friendly kind of guy.
- ♡ Weapons. It can be as a collector's item or decor for his pad. It's sexy and masculine.

Touch Me

It doesn't matter how much smoke you blow up Aries' ass, any form of flattery—lies and all—are taken in and fed right to his dick. After all, anyone who takes the time to feed his ego, even if it's just gas, is saying something. It says that someone is kissing up to him and that validates his belief that he's a fabulous and fuckable kind of guy. So, go for it and say whatever you think, real or not. As long as it sounds good and comes across moderately sincere, he'll soak it up. From there, he's yours for the taking—but again, remember the spaghetti theory. Timing is everything; so plot, maneuver yourself in place proper, and be ready to blast off.

Be inappropriate, he lives for that. Get dirty; he'll follow. Introduce him to new forms of sexual pleasure and you'll forever be his hero. By nature, an Aries man isn't hard to pleasure, but he's difficult to keep the interest of. Patience isn't something he comprehends. So use your imagination to stay free of the same ole sexual routines and challenge him to go for the gusto. Just make sure not to overwhelm, as he needs to feel like the leader. Sure, he'll play submissive for game, but will make it understood that it's a temporary role. He'll need the last word on the antics—so give it to him. Let him then show how his imagination can top yours and bring the sexcapades to the next level. It's this kind of fire that'll keep your passions going long and strong!

Ways to Heat Up Your Aries:

- ♡ Remember, his erogenous zone is his head; you can take this literally and metaphorically. Rub both of them and make him explode.
- ♡ Blow him in an elevator or a cab. He gets off easily on anything spontaneous and scandalous.
- ♡ Incite a fight with him and have makeup sex. It's the best kind he offers.
- ♡ Brag about his sexual prowess to others, and have him overhear it by "accident." The rush to his ego will be a potent aphrodisiac.
- ♡ Tie him up and make him your bitch. Losing control gets him hot—as long as it's not a regular routine you make him endure. As a novelty, he loves playing the slave.
- ♡ Use a timer in the bedroom and keep records on how fast or long it takes to climax. He loves breaking records.
- ♡ Tease him. Send him your undies soaked with some of your love juices, with a sexy photo of yourself and a letter describing the nasty things you want him to do to you.

Role-playing

Even in the most peaceful surroundings, Aries will bring in his suitcase of drama and throw it all around. He lives to stir things up, as nothing comes from placidness. This makes role-playing a perfect stage for him to let his thespian get as innovative and forceful as he likes. Aries thrives with roles that have distinct power positions—as he loves combat and blurring the lines between domination and submission. Of course, you can bet which role he prefers, but as you know, he's always open to new experiences, too. So, as long as you don't pigeonhole him, anything goes.

Cast of Characters:

♡ Soldier and prisoner of war. Any war-related fantasy works, as his sign rules it.

♡ Papa Bear and Goldilocks. It's that domination thing, mixed with innocence that'll get him hot every time.

♡ International businessman and pageant winner. Success and trophy pieces—what's not sexy about that? Nothing he'll be able to think of.

♡ Sheik and harem member. It's an exotic twist to the power idea.

♡ Boss and secretary. It's a classic power fantasy that can't go wrong with Aries.

♡ Explorer and a sexy local inhabitant. His dreams of going where no man has gone before.

♡ Prom night with his virgin date. It's all about being #1.

Taking the Bait

Underneath all that insanity he uses to cast a playboy image beats the heart of an old-fashioned boy with traditional values. While he might not submit to the established rules, he does look for the one he loves to follow those rules. Shockingly enough, Aries ideally is looking for a virgin to share forever with, despite having left a trail of used condoms all over town. It's because of this that many Aries do tend to marry while they are young. Of course, the vestal virgin fantasy tends to be just that for many, so don't get bent out of shape if you've got some miles on your tires. Obviously, when he falls in love all those rules go out the window. Remember, he loves to break the rules, even if they're his own.

In the face of love, he'll change everything. By nature, he's rude, unapologetic, self-centered, and completely off his rocker, and has a list of unrelenting needs. To get Aries to behave, only a few things will do the trick: if you're paying for his services (and it better be a large amount!), if you have blackmail on him, or if he's in love. Yes, he'll break out humility for love, but get it while he's hot, as this will subside in time, too, no matter how crazy he is for you. Consistency is not his thing, and it'll be up to you to know when to pull the leash and get him to obey. When he goes out of bounds and pisses you off, this will be the true test of his affections. If he can say he's sorry and admit fault, then know you've awakened a precious side to him—as he'd typically rather cut off his left ear than say that word. If he goes further to shower you with presents, forget even questioning his feelings—they're yours.

If you need more reassurance, you'll find it among his cronies. Like him, they'll be an opinionated bunch with an inability to hold back their feelings. With Aries having such a big mouth, they'll know every detail about you if he's smitten. Of course, this still won't mean you'll be home free, as he falls in and out of love quickly. Give this behavior several months to sink in and from there, start picking out your china patterns.

UNAUTHORIZED: ASTRAL AUTOPSY

Recognizing Fear

With the way he struts like a proud peacock, Aries would like you to believe he's fearless. Ha! He's obsessed by his fears and is either on a path to confront them or run from them. Fears are his little pills of adrenaline waiting to happen. Once he downs one, *bam!* One less thing in his life that can define him—and God knows he hates to be defined. Aries thinks of his fears as his ultimate to-do list, a never-ending series of tests that line the way to his destiny of invincibility or blocks him from really living. It's all just a matter of nature and nurture, which Aries manifests in yours: the daredevil or the drama queen chicken.

Main cause
Fear rules him, by way of inspiring or trapping him.

Immunizing His Fears:

- ♡ Compliment his looks periodically. A constant flow of flattery keeps him balanced.
- ♡ His pride is his most prized possession; guard it with your life. Defend his honor whenever necessary—even if you have to stage the moment, like getting rid of a friend you wanted to anyway and blaming it on him or her bad-mouthing him.
- ♡ Go to a horror movie and clutch on to him during the gory scenes. It'll make him feel like a "man."
- ♡ With any humbling situation for his ego, whether it's untying a really tight knot or asking for a raise, baby him. He'll instantly toughen up (someone with an Aries must have invented reverse psychology).
- ♡ In the presence of any scary unknown, offer to go first. Being second is a bigger fear for him.

Infecting Him with Fear:

- ♡ Whenever he gets mad, laugh at him. He'll be scared he's "lost it."
- ♡ He wants people to like him, so have him accidentally hear or find out that someone isn't that into him—or worse, have him find out someone only likes him because of you.
- ♡ Make your number show up as a private caller and every time the phone rings he'll freak wondering who's calling. Prey on his paranoia.

♡ He's a big fan of conspiracy theories; indulge him in more for your pleasure.

♡ Get him caught in a crowd; he'll get claustrophobic faster than you can count to ten.

Recognizing Anger

He's legendary for a short fuse and temper tantrums. Why? He's the brat of the zodiac and is too cocky for words. When he can't get his way, then comes his flood of frustrations. Unable to process this emotion as anything other than failure, he'll attempt to use anger to incite fear to seize control and what he believes is saving face. The more you resist, the more aggressive he'll become. Plus, he's relentless and won't give in until you implode or he really explodes. Either result is never a pretty sight and makes him out to look like an utter fool every time.

Main cause
Seeing that the world doesn't revolve around him.

Immunizing His Anger:

♡ Anger is a creative outlet for him, one he must express. Let it run its course, as everything he does is brief. Think of this act as his mental pooping.

♡ Always ask him about his day or about him—not like he needs an intro to start talking about himself, but he prefers it.

♡ Pee before you leave the house. He'll hate you if he has to stop after he gets going.

♡ Walk, talk, drive, and always act fast. Speed of any sort keeps him happy.

♡ Be more pissed off than he is. When faced with other's rage, he tends to want to add a calming effect to the situation. He's soothed with chaos.

Infecting Him with Anger:

- ♡ Aries hates other's self-centeredness—it takes the spotlight away from him. Talk about yourself incessantly and he'll hate you soon enough.
- ♡ Drive him nuts by making him wait by being late, and/or being slow—as in walking slowly, talking slowly, making decisions slowly, understanding what he's saying slowly, getting on an escalator slowly, changing the TV channels slowly and unrhythmically, etc.
- ♡ Don't be exuberantly thankful to him for gifts, dinner, etc. The grand gestures of thanks are why he does these things in the first place.
- ♡ Demasculinate him—like ask someone else to open the ketchup bottle instead of him. He'll burn with jealousy.
- ♡ Everything is a competition and he expects everyone to be as aggressive as him, even everyday things like hailing a cab. Be too polite and let others take the first cab; at a crowded bar, be passive about getting the bartender's attention—things of that nature make him mad.

Recognizing Sadness

He's not half-assed about anything, least of all sorrow. When it comes to being down in the dumps, Aries does it with all the fanfare most reserve for a state funeral. He knows how to do tragic, taking the term "emotional vampire" to new levels. However, sorrow can also be the feeling he's most private about, as he works so hard to project his image of perfection—so tread lightly if he lets you onto this ground, as the foundation is very delicate.

Main cause
Drama isn't effective without sorrow.

Immunizing His Sadness:

- ♡ Get sad with him. With two, it's officially a tragedy; he'll bounce back by taking charge.
- ♡ Periodically ask him the meaning of a word or defer to him for information. Being made to feel like an authority is essential to his maintenance.
- ♡ Set up a competition and let him win—even dumb things like, "Last one up is a rotten egg." No victory is too small.
- ♡ Take him out in public. His "all is perfect" façade goes up as soon as he enters the world.
- ♡ Buy him something. Money always cheers him up—the more lavish, the more effective.

Infecting Him with Sorrow:

- ♡ Make him feel old. He's all about being energetic and youthful; take this away and create misery.
- ♡ For your birthday or a holiday, coo over a gift you got from someone else as your favorite. If his isn't the best, it's endless pain.
- ♡ Seek his advice, but be sly in letting him know he's not the first person you asked. Like once he gives his advice, say, "Oh so-and-so said . . ." This will make him feel silently inferior, even if you called your shrink first.
- ♡ Screen his call. If he's not a priority, he'll wilt a little every time he hears another ring.
- ♡ Let him know others think he's selfish. This will rock his world, as he's under the delusion he's so selfless.

Recognizing Trust

Aries' suspicious nature makes it hard for him to trust anyone, unless you're his subordinate. Even so, he'll only give you so much trust and it'll be in the form of commands, because he only relies on people who know their place in his presence, deeming everyone else a moron or a threat. However, relying on someone and trusting him or her has a dividing line, which he keeps gray on purpose. Preferring to keep everyone at a distance, he likes to think he's so self-reliant that he can maintain everyone at a disposable level. For those who fall through the cracks, he's just waiting for them to mess up.

Main cause
He's the best, so who else can he turn to?

Immunizing Him With Trust:

♡ His cocky defenses are annoying, but if you can keep loyal with him through time, that'll be your ticket to his trust.

♡ Give him something of value that's yours (like a family heirloom) and show your trust first; he'll be open to following.

♡ Borrow money from him and pay back quickly without asking. His money is the only thing he trusts. Show you respect it; win his admiration.

♡ Call him on his lies, which he'll periodically do (or at least exaggerate the truth), as not taking his shit wins his respect, aka trust.

♡ Buy into his conspiracy theories—like avoiding certain topics while talking on a cell phone and live in a state of paranoia he thinks exists.

Infecting His Trust:

♡ Be competitive with your professional aspirations, even if you're in different fields. The fact that you're trying to outshine his accomplishments will make him cringe. After all, you can't trust the enemy.

♡ Act cautious. Like reducing your speed when approaching a yellow light instead of speeding up to pass. If you don't take risks, he won't understand you, let alone trust you.

♡ Split a restaurant or bar bill 50/50 even though you ordered more, but disregard that fact. He'll consider this suspicious behavior.

♡ Give out your zip code to cashiers openly, without question. He can't trust anyone who's not as neurotic as him.

♡ Have at least one of his friends like you as much as they like him. Have them call you instead of him to confirm plans. Even if this happens once, it'll make him feel threatened eternally.

Recognizing Motivation

Aries is driven by his ego. Having a plethora of inferiority complexes, he's out to prove he's the biggest, baddest, and best. Being a victim to the machismo stereotype in one form or another, undermining his is a surefire way to goad him into action. All you need to do is make a suggestion that makes him feel he has to prove himself; add a competitive element and he'll bring it. As for keeping him motivated, realize poor follow-through is his curse. However, if you can define or offer a carrot at the end of the stick, then you might have him going to the end.

Main cause

He was born with a fire under this ass, just no map with where to go with it.

Immunizing His Motivation:

♡ Refuse to follow. He may be independent and all, but without someone who obeys, he can't lead and what's the point, unless he's in charge?

♡ In any activity, get someone who's more of a pro than him involved. He'd rather quit than submit to being second-fiddle.

♡ Make anything slow and repetitious and he'll fall asleep.

♡ Set up anything for the long term. His impatience is too powerful to tame.

♡ Always be ready with many other options. In the face of choices, he can get scattered and paralyzed.

Infecting His Motivation:

♡ If he leaves an idea of his unused that you'd like to see him take action on, mention you'll suggest it to someone else. He'll jump to his feet to accomplish the goal, because he'd hate someone else claiming his glory.

♡ Aries loves trying new things. Offer up any adventure that deals with the unexplored and/or a bit of danger and there's no stopping him.

♡ Attach coolness points to something you want him to do or paint it as a way for him to gain popularity.

♡ Ultimatums make him unresponsive, but challenge always gets his attention. Double dog dare him, it works every time.

♡ Tell him, "If you do it, I'll do it," or take the lead role yourself. Whatever the situation you find yourself in he'll go into action if the head role is part of the deal or if he can seize it from someone else. Being #1 in any sense is his inspiration.

DESTINATION: DUMPSVILLE

Celestial Voodoo on You

Aries has no attention span and his turnover rate is high. Unless you can keep him constantly enthralled and on his toes by spinning out new talents every seventy-two hours, like being able to eat fire and suck cock, then expect your exit to be imminent. Aries likes things now. He gets off on peeling the wrapper more than he does on eating the candy and goes through dates like underwear—and even so, his underwear may get more soiled than you. Being that he's quick to move on, you may not even know he's gone by the time he's gone. He cuts things off fast and abruptly. One day he'll be madly in love with you, the next you'll get his breakup memo. Typically, this memo is something short, sweet, and completely nonpersonal. The reality is that long-term anything leaves him claustrophobic. When anything starts to get a bit familiar, Aries considers his options. If it's more exciting to find something new than fix something old, then he's out the door.

Not to say there's no heartbreak for Aries, but generally his affairs are so brief that no one ever has any time to really bond—making it almost acceptable that he can bid his adieu via e-mail, voice mail, or text message. If your tryst lasted longer than a few sessions of hot sex and several personal facts shared, then he might offer his more valiant side of breaking up—which tends to be just as annoying. It entails granting himself an overblown idea of importance to you and making a long and highly ridiculous self-righteous exit speech recited like he's some high-ranking military official. At least with this, it'll make it blaringly obvious why you'll want to be done with him, too.

Of course, the worst is Aries trying to get out of a "serious" relationship, as he's clumsy and arrogant and can't communicate his emotions effectively because he can't handle personal pressure to save his life. In a constant struggle with this ego and inferiorities, he gets messy when given any power—making it all about him, not you or your relationship. In this situation, he'll create more drama than necessary. If you concede and offer up compassion, that'll infuriate him just the same—as he'll feel undermined. Unless he can call all the shots and play hero, he's never happy. Of course, no one in their right mind will allow him that and that's why an Aries' breakup is more like a smash up. Fortunately for you, being that he's so haughty, chances are in your favor that it's his psyche that deto nates, rather than yours, and at that point you'll be too exhausted to even care.

. . . And Other Signs He Hates You

Aries hates without mixed messages. When an Aries hates you, you know it. He thrives with enemies to direct his anger toward and gets off acting like the bully in a schoolyard, flexing his power like it's a masturbatory exhilaration. He's rude, obnoxious, and arrogant and will get in your face with unapologetic behavior that can be embarrassing—embarrassing for him that is. Think of all those crazy over-the-top machismo maniacs and you'll get Aries in his prime hate mode: talking loudly, spewing off anything to humiliate you, and dishing out whatever low blow he's got.

The thing to keep in mind, though, is that he's got a short attention span. While you may be the main object of his hate for a set time, usually with his superior attitude his disdain will soon be directed toward someone new. If you want your time to pass as his public enemy #1, all you have to do is stick it out. His time is precious and typically he'll retreat when he gets bored calling you the same names. Once you get swept aside, you can join the legions of friends he has left behind for all sorts of random reasons. You can also take comfort in the fact that all his loyal constituents are usually a few steps from being hated, too. To him, being a leader is about controlling emotions and being independent. Ridiculous, yes, you'll know it, but him, clueless. Oh well.

Beating Him to the Punch

Aries is usually so oblivious to anyone's feelings but his own that he'll typically be blindsided when getting dumped. However, getting him all excited can be to your detriment. So, when you're ready to cut the cord, realize you have to do some prep work to achieve the maximum results—or expect his charismatic-to-psychotic freak to emerge or the charming negotiator who will want to lure you back to dump you. What you're striving for is a nice clean break, which he'll chivalrously adhere to if you set your plans in motion early on, somewhat like reverse foreplay. To begin, start to numb him down. Ignore him and only want to talk about yourself. If this goes on for a while, he'll dump you in no time—so don't do this too long. A weekend will be fine.

Next, bore him to tears. Act too tired to do anything, especially sex, and then be unenthused about his ideas. Cling to him more than necessary and be too dependent—over the silliest things too. Instead of wondering what's wrong with you, he'll be concerned about his own entertainment. Then when you tell him you would like to end things, give him the humbling speech of how he deserves so much better and all that crap. By making him sleepy and then feeding his ego a bit, he'll give you what you want peacefully. If you try to go about it any other way, like cutting him off quick and messing with his pride, then you're asking for trouble. Unless you like migraines, going this nonevasive route is the surefire way to get yourself out intact.

Ridding Yourself of Aries with Minimal Scarring:

- ♡ Be the dead-weight bottom in bed one too many times.
- ♡ Insult him in public. Better yet, get his friends to laugh at him—even if it's in jest, it can be deadly if you touch too close to his ego.
- ♡ Write a letter and bolt. Sometimes it's just about saving yourself.
- ♡ Be overly demanding about everything. No one is his boss but him.

♡ Be better than him at anything that involves competition or being compared. This could be anything from board games, sports, or to how much money you make. If you show him up in too many categories, he'll take it personally and have to leave you behind.

♡ Become too complicated with problems of your own and stress financial issues. His wallet is the last place where he'll want to dig for help.

♡ Let yourself go when you're in public together. His vanity will save you!

Kick, Drop, and Kill

He's hardcore, knows how to push buttons, and will repeatedly do it until you're worn thin. The pain and aggression felt under Aries' ego is like no other and maneuvering away unscathed requires the mental agility of an escape artist. However, once free from his clutches, your dexterity to handle pressure soars and you'll officially earn your stripes in the boot camp of love.

The fact is this guy can be a lunatic and incredibly unaccountable for his irrational actions. The thing is, though, these qualities that have driven you to the brink of insanity are the same ones that made you fall for him in the first place. Unwittingly, this makes him a round-trip adventure in which you see the light and dark side to all that's fun, fearless, aggressive, arrogant, charming, cool, psychotic, explosive, unsuspectingly kind, spontaneous, and of course, perpetually horny. Yeah, it was a dirty job loving him, but hell, somebody had to do it.

WANTED: TAURUS

BORN: APRIL 20—MAY 22

 Couch-bound sensualist with slow reaction time. Chronically adverse to change and most likely found where you last left him. Gets erect from the scent of fried chicken.

BARE BASICS

How to Spot Him

No matter where you are—a riot or a picnic, look for the comfortable place to plant your ass and most likely there's where you'll encounter Taurus. Despite any wild energy that looms through the air, he's the eye of the storm—lounging about with his big ole cow eyes, classic clean looks, sturdy physique, and no-frills style. There's comfort in his energy, like a bowl of mashed potatoes on a cold and damp day that lures the prospects in with a welcoming approach.

Yes, Taurus has got a sturdy way about him, and no matter if he's preppy or punk, he looks destined to be a soccer dad. Usually found in a pack of male accomplices, Taurus isn't one of those boys who seek out trouble. He just likes being around the action and deriving all the benefits of such. He'll be the one with his ass planted down, beer in hand and looking content. Like everything he does, being social is a spectator sport. After all, his official role is as the nice guy. Although this is sometimes to his detriment, as he tends to get stuck as the wingman to his horny and crass friends. However, it's not that he minds, he loves conversation and really getting to know who people are. Plus, it suits him fine to be the comforting stranger, as he's not overly aggressive; a slow pace to courting suits him fine.

Not to say he takes what he gets, no way. As represented by the bull, when he does see something or someone who brings out his hunger, he's relentless about what he desires (even if sometimes it's just obsessing on his unrequited passion). Typically, he uses kindness to work his way into the heart of his intended. Then, once he knows the odds are in his favor, he'll go full force with the romance. After all, he's a sensualist, ruled by the love side of Venus, making him a fool for it. He lives by his five senses and is hedonistically connected to his body, always giving his lovers a wooing worth remembering. You bet he'll bring flowers, ensure reservations at the most divine restaurants, and get you to swoon in perfect timing to his extending arm ready to grab you with one fell swoop.

Taurus is programmed to strive for absolute love, comfort, and pleasure, and he takes it seriously. When it comes to love or even lust, he's all heart—so know he's sincere as he sits there at the edge of his seat gazing upon you, hanging on your every word and making you feel like the most delicately beautiful and soulful being he has ever encountered.

Key Features:

- ♡ A sturdy to stocky body type with a meaty and solid stature
- ♡ Big cow eyes that exude innocence
- ♡ A strong and/or long neck
- ♡ An unshaven look or the type prone to growing a beard
- ♡ A plain and casual style of dress
- ♡ A pleasant speaking voice
- ♡ A calm and grounding energy about him

Seducing Him into Your Boudoir

Taurus man doesn't play to fuck around. He's a relationship guy who rarely approaches sex as a recreational sport with rotating players on his team. Although he's competitive, his goal is finding true love. His prize: nesting mode, as comfort is what he craves. The macho phase of getting notches on his belt, due to ego or peer pressure, is usually short. The truth is that he's traditionally monogamous and territorial.

He wants a connection that's sweet, sexy, loving, and all his. Vying for this role means being on this wavelength and effectively intoxicating him through his senses—as that's how he operates. Taurus looks at his prospects from all angles, like he's buying a fine piece of china. To him, each conquest is a possible mate for life, so he's very careful and examines compatibility on many levels. He doesn't want someone he can screw but can't get mushy with or bring home to his family. So, step #1: provide warm conversation about your career, family, and hobbies. Your stability factor will matter. Sure, it sounds a bit like a job interview, but this is how he functions—logically and sensibly. After he knows he's attracted to you, body and mind, score extra points in the domestic skills category.

He gets turned on by the whole idea of being a couple, so understand Taurus is examining you for culinary capabilities, money management prowess, and kid-friendly quotient—that perfect 2.3 family statistic and some. Even if he isn't the most traditional Taurus, he'll appreciate this homey form of seduction about you. Stability is his thing, and his lovers need to be able to kick back on the couch, eat a bag of chips, and shoot the shit in front of a TV or whatever low-key activity old married couples do—as that's what he idealizes, the comfort of being with you. No, this isn't for everyone, but he's quite specific about looking for someone to melt into and turn into an even bigger and better blob that oozes with love.

Loving Him in the Boudoir

Set your time aside, because when it comes to sex, he's no in-and-out job. When Taurus is in the sack, he's there to stay—and most likely, the foreplay began even before the touching. When near you, he's taking in all of you: the scent of your hair, the suppleness of your skin, the slope of your lower back into your ass, the way you taste behind your ears, the sound of your voice when you call his name—everything!

He breaks you down piece by piece with all his five senses, as Taurus takes in his lovers absolutely and completely. He's not scared to commit. He knows what he likes and cares for what he loves. He's a thorough man and when he's says he's in, he's in. He's a man you call to get the job done right. So, expect full service when it comes to the "wining and dining" before, after, and during the chase. Taurus will give you great conversations, bond on several emotional levels, and whisk you away to romantic scenarios worthy of Harlequin covers.

Yes, the Taurian appetite for romance, sex, and all things physical is large! He's insatiable and once he likes the taste of something, he likes to chow down hard. He's an indulgent soul and there's no curbing his desires, so take advantage. Plus, he won't just give you generic screwing, he'll give you a full-body experience that'll integrate every inch of you and whatever other creative and sensual toys he's got up his sleeve all in the name of pleasure. He's a giver in bed, much more than most others in the zodiac, and he isn't doing it for his ego, either. To him, each escapade is a sexual masterpiece that is sculpted by its length of time, chemistry, and imagination— this is his pledge and the way he believes it needs to be.

MAKING HIM COME TO THE PALM OF YOUR HAND

Eye Candy

Don't let his practical and placid demeanor fool you. Under his basic cotton tees breathes a clotheshorse who is just as vain as he is hungry. While he isn't necessarily all about flash and pricey labels, he is about quality and holding himself with class—which means he's looking for a match set when it comes to his Honey's style. He wants a lover with a smart look who is sexy in a sensual way, but subtle enough to be able to go anywhere and fit in. He likes durable fashion, styles that can be mixed and matched and worn for a variety of occasions. In a nutshell, he likes enduring basics, just the way he prefers his lovers.

Stylin' Seduction:

- ♡ Rich earthy colors, such as hunter green, brown, and dark red. Those are shades he's soothed by.
- ♡ Velvet, silk, satin—fabrics pleasing to the touch. He loves using his five senses, and touch is one of his favorites.
- ♡ Fitted styles that are professional and polished looking. He likes a tailored look, but not uptight—something classic.
- ♡ Flower and nature prints, as long as they're subtle and tasteful. He's totally into the nature thing.
- ♡ Clothes you might wear on a camping trip. Not that you need to sport this look every day, but he does have a soft spot for a sexy outdoorsy look.
- ♡ Quality matters. He's the type to check the seams, making sure the pieces are well made. His logic: If you adorn yourself with clothes of poor workmanship, you might also cut corners with the quality of love you give.

♡ Thick and natural-flowing hair. Forget the products; he's all about running his fingers through your hair and taking in its natural scent.

Tasty Treats

Food

Anorexics need not apply. Food is Taurus' epicenter. He most likely will be armed with a fabulous culinary skill all his own, but rest assured anyone who knows their way around a kitchen has got an easy in to his affections. His heart is his stomach, and if he's not fed right, nothing goes right. Not one to fill up on salad, he's a meat-and-potatoes kind of man and loves a good meal that sticks to his ribs. You better believe it, like everything that he consumes; he wants it to be rich, hearty, and filling. He wants substance, not just suste-nance. Give this to him and he'll be putty in your hands.

Erotic Eats:

♡ Restaurants with hearty foods, using lots of sauces and gravies. Steakhouses are perfect. Also, any place that serves things like stews, goulashes, chili, or fondues will hit the spot.

♡ A place with a homey atmosphere where he can really chow down and at reasonable prices. He's got a practicality thing about him, too.

♡ Deep-fried food joints. He loves grease!

♡ Gourmet dining. Taurus is the sign of sensuality, so fine din-ing is his idea of romance. Plus, being that he's typically so no-nonsense, anything deemed expensive will turn him on.

♡ Ethnic eateries. French, German, and American are prime choices. They all generally have a heaviness to the textures to their food—giving him that filling feeling he adores.

♡ Dinner cooked by you or have him cook you dinner. Home is his preferred place to be; add food to the mix and you're just that much closer to the boudoir and the nesting mode he so craves.

♡ Pastries. Taurus loves dessert. It's the finale of any proper dining experience. Know good dessert spots and your night could only get sweeter.

Movies

Taurus is a total cinemaphile. He can't resist assaulting his emotional sensors while sitting on his ass, with food in hand and possibly a little of you in the other. It's a whole experience that's catered for his energy level. As for genres that pique his interest: movies with heart. Yes, he's secure enough in his masculinity to go see a tearjerker and even shed a tear or two, but the films must have plot and some artistic merit. You know it, movies with some meat!

Cinematic Foreplay:

♡ Award-winning movies. Whether it's Oscar or some festival, films with any sort of critical "stamp of approval" are good with him.

♡ Classics, including old black-and-white or silent movies. He's an old-fashioned kind of guy.

♡ Romance—comedies or drama. Most Taurians are suckers for Merchant Ivory–type flicks.

♡ Drama: tearjerkers, melodramas, and coming-of-age tales. He's a big old sap under it all.

♡ Epic stories. He's got all the patience in the world to watch a deep and heavy plot play out.

♡ Films involving food. Anything involving food captures his imagination.

♡ Movies with pretty cinematography. Again, his senses need to be pleased.

Dating Ideas

Taurians are a mixed bag of surprises. He can be found at two extremes: a total couch potato or a fitness freak. He's got both in him and is rarely in between. However, those two extremes can be a cause and effect. When he wants something, he works like a fiend to get it, but once he commits, he can lull in the comfort zone. So, while he's in the impressing phases of his courtship, you might wonder what this talk about being lazy is all about. Realize many a Taurus, once he's pledged his undying love, will go into a couch-potato coma. It's been known to happen time and time again, so it's essential to work his keister to the max with activities that'll inspire him to keep active.

Playful Planning:

♡ Bowling. It doesn't take much effort and there's lots of beer around; he'll love it.

♡ Race-car events or any fast-paced sports. Although he's no speed demon, he likes being a spectator to adrenaline— pumping excitement. It's a vicarious thing.

♡ Nature. Most Taurians dig exercising outside: hiking, cycling, or Rollerblading are ideal.

♡ Music, dance, theater, or other artistic performances. He's ruled by Venus, endowing him with an appreciation for the arts.

♡ Food-related events, such as festivals, cooking class, or venturing on some culinary adventure, like wine tasting. His tongue is one of his favorite muscles to use.

♡ Museums and art exhibitions, perfect for slow strolling and conversation. He has a soft spot for culture, even if it isn't obviously apparent.

♡ Homeward-bound dates, like dinner and a movie. He's a gentleman and won't put the moves on you, unless you give the green light.

Sound Seduction

Conversation

His energy is smooth, easygoing, and kindhearted — the type of guy to languish about on a Sunday afternoon and share your innermost secrets with. He's not self-centered, either, and really does want to hear what's on your mind. In fact, Taurus is one of the best listeners out there. However, if you want to turn this around, there could be some problems, as he doesn't enjoy being in the spotlight. Sure, he'll talk, but he's typically a man of few words. His preferred way is listening and showing how he feels through his actions. So, when it comes to cracking open his mind, stick to the definite things about him—things he can solidly speak of and he'll gladly let you in.

Icebreakers:

♡ Ask him about his favorite foods and his reasons why. Talking about food is an art unto itself for Taurus.

♡ Test his romance quotient. What's his idea of a perfect weekend getaway?

♡ Discuss books. He's a bookworm and can be never-ending with recommendations.

♡ Bring up his childhood and family—all Taurians are into them. Whether it's absolute love or hate, he'll love blabbering on and on about them.

♡ Talk about past relationships. While this would be a no-no for some, this man loves talking about love-related topics. He's not scared to share his mistakes, either.

♡ Ask him questions that deal with his stability factor—such as what car does he drive? Where does he live? Does he own or rent? It's a safe conversation that'll loosen him up, as he prides himself on having answers for these kinds of questions.

♡ I love him share his complaints. Taurus usually holds a lot in because no one ever asks. Be the one to go there and find out what pisses him off and you'll wonder how to ever shut him up!

Music

Next to his cupboards, his CD collection is the next most bountiful possession. Music is the way Taurus can best explain his feelings and thoughts. He's the sign most likely to express himself with a mix CD to show his affections. Being a master DJ, he knows how to translate his soul into a musical combination that resonates in you deeper than words. His music tastes are large and vast and he's got a sound for every mood and thought. He'll be into the hard stuff, the soft stuff, and anything that offers a deep and majestic experience that can transport body and mind.

Mood Makers:

♡ Soulful funk and/or R&B. A smooth vibe appeals to his sense of calm.

♡ Classic or heavy rock. If it's got a good hook, put it on.

♡ House music. Anything he can easily groove with works.

♡ American popular music (e.g., Frank Sinatra). Taurians usually have pleasant singing voices and love belting it out with other singers.

♡ Acoustic/folk. It'll awaken his sensitive side.

♡ Bossa nova. Its chill romantic vibe will speak to him.

♡ Opera. It's highbrow and overwhelming, the filet mignon of music—casting a romantic mood he won't be able to refuse.

Gifts

Every aspect of gift giving is important to Taurus. While others may just throw something in a bag, Taurus thinks it crass. Presentation matters, as he considers the entire process of gift giving a theatrical gesture. He pays attention to everything: the wrapping, the timing, the mood you created, and of course, the object of your affections. If you present well, it won't even matter what's in the box.

Boxed Treats:

- ♡ Gadgets for every day. Something for his kitchen, computer, or bathing needs are always pleasers. Practical is his taste.
- ♡ Anything edible. Whether it's a thong made of a flank steak in your size or his favorite cheese, he'll love it!
- ♡ A framed photo from a sentimental moment you both shared. He'll feel your love from it forever.
- ♡ Gift certificates from a music store. It's a gift that can never go wrong with this avid music lover.
- ♡ Wine. He's usually a connoisseur and will always offer to drink it with you. Double bonus!
- ♡ Video games. A guy who loves sitting around this much likes having a purpose; like, say, virtually saving the world.
- ♡ Clothes. Sure, it's unromantic and unexciting, but it's these little mothering gifts that'll go a long way with him.

Touch Me

Taurus is Mr. Lover-Man. He gives new standards to the idea of marathon sex because he can go way past the finish line, breaking every record in the book. He's got so much stamina that you better have a bunch of kinky ideas to keep the excitement climaxing—as he scores high in technique but low in artistic merit. Sure, he can go all night and give it good, with much consistency. However, his fatal flaw is he can be a one-trick pony. He likes routine and once he finds the way to giving you the ultimate orgasm, he'll be a repeat offender, using the same moves over and over again, until you go dry. So be prepared to change it up and avoid the rut, which can eventually lead to boredom. Understand, like a pot roast in the oven, he needs to be turned round and round to have the taste be at its prime.

To get extra-juicy flavor and non-stop heart-pounding banging, know his stimulation is at its peak if the environment is right—which means thinking ahead. He's at his best with ambiance, and the bedroom is where he's at his highest comfort level. There he's free to let loose all his sensors to grope for titillation. So, light the aromatherapy candles; break out the twelve-hundred-thread-count bedsheets, massage oils, body paints, whip cream, and sexy lingerie; pour the wine; and turn on the sultry sexathon music, because you'll need a five-ring sensory circus to bring out his most insatiable love animal and the ultimate satisfaction.

However, despite all the accoutrements you can toss into the scene, there's one aspect that's irreplaceable when it comes to getting Taurus to turn into a triple-threat vibrating drilling machine—and that's love. He thrives on satisfying and making his lovers swoon with desire for him and only him—and this is usually only the case when he's in love. With love, he's at his most comfortable, as that's the key word in getting him to dazzle you in the sack. After all, he doesn't want to know all the work he's putting into learning your body, and what makes you come will go to waste after a few shots of love juice and snoozy times. No way, he's all about the buildup and that takes time. So be glad for this, as his insistence on upholding the traditional pillars of romance will make you understand what it's like to be appreciated as a work of art.

Ways to Heat Up Your Taurus:

♡ Remember that his neck and throat are his astral g-spots, so run your hands here while making out.

♡ Make your body a sensorium of things to touch, smell, taste, etc. Example: velvet thongs and chocolate body paint.

♡ His three favorite things are sex, money, and food. Jump him at a drive-in ATM after he makes a big deposit or after a food pickup. Just make sure you don't make him choose between you and the food; you might get insulted with his decision.

♡ Give him a full-body massage with or without oil and ask for the same. Either way, he'll oblige kindly and then need to fuck you after. For added kink, use a blindfold.

♡ Rub his earlobes; no Taurus man can resist this!

♡ Greet him at the door with nothing on but an apron and then do him on the kitchen floor. It's a classic Taurus sex fantasy.

♡ Stick food into your orifices and have him eat it out—any and most orifices will do, but perhaps not the nose; that may be too gross for him.

Role-playing

He's a good-natured plaything who will do anything for his lover. If dressing up and changing identities is what you like, count him in. The thing, though, Taurus isn't so much into character development as he's scene driven—better at playing into an ambiance than about going inside to bring out a new persona. Start slow and then pick up the pace. Characters he'll play best will lean toward the ordinary on the outside, eccentric on the inside. Once he eases in, move him slowly into more complex scenarios. In no time, he'll be out buying costumes and making soundtracks for your tawdry theatrics.

Cast of Characters:

- ♡ Hotel maid and traveling businessman. A good starter fantasy to get his feet wet.
- ♡ Plumber/electrician and house caller. He'll make the most of using props.
- ♡ Artist and muse. His sign is ruled by Venus, the arts planet, making this an easy role for him to do.
- ♡ Chef and an erotic piece of pastry. Anything with food will bring out his most sensual side.
- ♡ A pioneer couple on the first night in their log cabin. The rusticness will turn him on.
- ♡ Prehistoric beings using only their five senses to communicate. He's the most sensual of the zodiac; this will put the focus on his true talents.
- ♡ Rodeo star and bar floozy. Taurians all have a "down-home" kind of guy in him.

Taking the Bait

Taurus love feels like a big ole bear hug. It takes you over completely and there's no escaping it. Expect to be overwhelmed with a secure and blissful sensation, making you warm and tingly in all the right spots. Being with him is much like putting on a warm and dry pair of socks after a rainstorm, a reassuring feeling made apparent by his sweet acts of kindness and consideration that'll have you all in a daze. Forget having to look for clues of his affection, as his dedication is undeniable. Taurus is not fooling around and when he's truly in love, he goes all out.

For one thing, in love, he's no longer shy and has no troubles going right into the "we" mode. He thrives best in a committed situation, as Taurus likes setting down roots and getting comfortable. At first, you'll love having him around because he really works on making

an effort to help you out and be part of your life. He'll perform duti-
ful acts of appreciation—the grandest gestures will be involving
food, no doubt. Yes, his courtship is filled with sweetness and sublime fantasies of future bliss. It'll have you wondering, Why was it
that easy? There has to be a hitch, right?

Right.

With Taurus, he'll get you in the back end, saving the hard part
after you've already signed on. You better believe it, once Taurus
has taken the bait and integrated himself into your life, you become
his foundation and he settles in. In no time, his ass is on your couch
as a human tumor. It starts slowly, as nights to cuddle with him that
you find so sweet will slowly turn into nights with him laid out with
the remote control in one hand, a beer can in the other, and food
stains on his shirt. It's hardly romantic or even very attractive when
he gets this mushy.

With Taurus, he'll consider his work done after commitment and
this is why he loves it so. Once he seals the deal, he can reap the
rewards. Not to say he loses all his romantic mojo, but he'll use it
sparingly. This then forces your hand and brain to understand one
thing: Keeping up your dreamy love wonderland that he's painted
requires that you become the keeper of the flame—the flame that
you have to hold under his ass every so often to keep the action
happening throughout your relationship. You may have to get stern,
creatively letting him know that there's a level of maintenance and
that there's more than comfort, especially his. As long as you're prepared for this change of events, as it takes pure grit to keep this man
at his best, things can remain beautiful. Keep him inspired with sensual fun and he'll stay with you in a permanent honeymoon mode.

UNAUTHORIZED: ASTRAL AUTOPSY

Recognizing Fear

Change freaks him out. Taurus likes to know where he is, what's around him, and who he's with. Security is where he flourishes, and dragging him to the great unknown messes his mind. Routine is his friend, and nailing one has been an ongoing lifelong process—and it's not work he'd want to necessarily redo either. However, it's not that he won't rise to the occasion if his life called for it, but he doesn't easily or pleasantly stray far from his norm.

Main cause
Having to go out of his comfort zone.

Immunizing His Fears:

♡ When going out, be prepared to do most of the talking. He's reserved with his words and prefers being out of the spotlight.

♡ Stick to going to the same places to eat, shop, etc. Familiarity soothes him.

♡ Plan ahead and move at a slow pace. Being rushed scares him.

♡ Always keep food on you, like candy, chips, or a sandwich. It's an effective pacifier.

♡ Make decisions decisively and be ready to lead. He has no ego issues with being a follower.

Infecting Him with Fear:

♡ He's into being punctual, when heading somewhere, like a movie. Freak him out by telling him you got the movie time wrong or your watch died and you could be late.

- ♡ Go on a long journey with no provisions stocked away or access to any.
- ♡ Keep him busy and constantly social. Vegging is his staple, without it he can lose it.
- ♡ Constantly change your look. He'll get paranoid that you're looking for change and worry you'll soon dump his ass.
- ♡ Eat off his plate without asking. He's super territorial about food and adhering to proper dining manners.

Recognizing Anger

He's famous for his patience and infamous for his insane anger. He doesn't readily lose it, which misleads people into thinking he's so understanding. He breaks out the anger only when his generous benefit of the doubt has worn thin—and once that line is crossed, he doesn't come back. If his patience has been ignored or he finally realizes he's been duped into becoming a total doormat, he answers with rage. As tolerant as he can be is how angry he can get, giving his bull symbol a new meaning as he goes into fighter mode, charging forward with only one thing on his mind: attack and destroy.

Main cause
His Mr.-Nice-Guy routine backfires.

Immunizing His Anger:

- ♡ If you like the same TV shows as him, this will make his life all that easier.
- ♡ Appreciate his traditions, as they're sacred to him.
- ♡ Give him lots of time to make up his mind.
- ♡ Ask him to confirm facts. Taurus has a complex about being stupid; if you defer to his mind it'll bring him eternal happiness.

♡ Be aware and appreciative of the little things he does for you, like the domestic duties he'll take on or the patience he provides. If you do this, you can do no wrong in his eyes.

Infecting Him with Anger:

♡ Overspend cash on needless items. He hates impractical spending.

♡ Have poor manners in public, like burping and farting. He'll laugh the first few times, but once you cross the line he'll want to dump you.

♡ Waste your food. This will drives him nuts. Of course, being wasteful in general will bug him—like use too much toilet paper, lots of soap, too many napkins, etc.

♡ Never let him taste what you order when you eat out, even after he asks how it is.

♡ Don't take this question seriously, "What do you want for dinner?"

Recognizing Sadness

There's no way to avoid depression when you allow yourself to turn into a sloth—and that's the conundrum that is Taurus. He lives for his comforts, often ODing on it and then winds up being uninspired and turning into one sad mess of lumpy flesh that has no clue how to get back on track. Sure, he can happily thrive in this rut for longer than most, but life without change does catch up to him.

Main cause
Too much of a good thing.

Immunizing His Sadness:

- ♡ Get jealous every so often, so he'll know he's loved
- ♡ Keep aspirin on you. He's prone to headaches and will be touched you're thinking about his comfort.
- ♡ Get him to express himself artistically. He's creative and he needs to be reminded of that.
- ♡ Play to his masochistic side; whip his ass with some tough love and jog his brain back into positivity.
- ♡ Cook for him. Again, food is the answer to most questions you can have about this man.

Infecting Him with Sorrow:

- ♡ Drop a subtle hint he needs to work out more; he has major body issues, prey upon them.
- ♡ Do something like drink wine with a straw; such déclassé behavior will cause him to get sad that he has to dump you.
- ♡ Hint to him that someone, a stranger (waitress, bartender, toll booth worker, etc.) doesn't like him, the original die-hard people pleaser. One misconstrued comment is all you need to take him down.
- ♡ Spend less money on his birthday present than he did on yours.
- ♡ Tell him you don't like being touched when you sleep. Spooning is his thing.

Recognizing Trust

He hates drama. Taurus lives to be consistently content and keeps an at-your-honor policy—meaning he's a trusting soul who goes with the flow. Sure, he gets that the world has its fair share of assholes, but his attitude is innocent until proven guilty. He's a "cross that bridge when you get there" kind of guy and really doesn't get why people would go out of their way to be jerks—so he won't go out of his way trying to find the worst in people, either. It's this attitude that crowns Taurus as the most well-adjusted in the zodiac.

Main cause
Trust makes comfort so much easier.

Immunizing Him with Trust:

- ♡ Be domestically inclined. The more skilled you are around the house, the more wholesome he'll think of you.
- ♡ Stick to him like glue. Nothing says trust like co-dependence!
- ♡ Be cautious with your money, like be constantly saving and ensuring your security.
- ♡ Keep him numb with comfort—aka well fed and sexually satisfied and he'll never suspect anything wrong anywhere. Touch him a lot; physical affection is essential to his comfort.
- ♡ Be punctual. How you respect people's time is a direct correlation to your character.

Infecting His Sense of Trust:

- ♡ Be a fickle eater. Your relationships with food matters to him.
- ♡ Be a last-minute person. Scramble about until the last minute and accidentally leave things behind. Be chaotic and he'll never get on your wavelength.
- ♡ Change your opinions with whomever you're with, but with little things. For example: Tell him Geneva is your favorite city in Europe. Then drop that your favorite city is Paris when talking to one of his friends.
- ♡ Don't keep a schedule, pay bills at the zero hour, laugh when you're careless, and never talk about the future. Be a "here and now" person.
- ♡ Make everything you do a competition. He won't trust you if he constantly feels he has to prove himself.

Recognizing Motivation

Taurus doesn't readily like to stray from his shtick. This typically means languishing in a home with food, friends, and family surrounding him in a state of perpetual ease during his free time and then working like a maniac every other minute. Getting Taurus to move his ass in a different direction is his Achilles' heel, as he's stubborn and complacent. However, motion is a fact of life he has to keep up and so he does.

Main cause
He's got responsibilities; therefore he has to get off his ass.

Immunizing His Motivation:

♡ Prop him up with fluffy pillows on a broken-in couch, place a remote nearby, and have snacks strewn all around him. He won't go anywhere when he's so comfortable.

♡ He'll do anything to save a dime. Paint anything to be expensive and he'll bail.

♡ Starve him and drain him of any energy. His blood sugar drops faster than everyone else—so he'll tell you.

♡ Wait until the pressure hits the zero hour to give him choices. He'd rather bow out than burst a blood vessel thinking fast.

♡ Have too many cooks in the kitchen. Anywhere there's too many loud opinions swirling about will close him up.

Infecting Him with Motivation:

♡ Play the victim. He won't hesitate to do anything for his loved ones, especially when they are feeling down and out.

♡ Change the furniture around and/or repaint the room. You might not be able to change Taurus, but you can change what's around him. While adapting, he'll change whatever else he needs to about himself, too. He likes doing things in blocks.

♡ Bribery. He loves money and will do anything for more of it.
♡ Put him to a stamina test. He loves to show his endurance. For example: Get him to a gym and watch him overwork himself to keep up with the hard bodies there.
♡ Pump him up with sugar and he'll get so antsy he'll have to get off his ass.

DESTINATION: DUMPSVILLE

Celestial Voodoo on You

You'd have to be in a coma to miss a Taurus wanting to dump you. He's stubborn and refuses to give in easy. He'll try every which way to make a situation work, even when there's only a minuscule amount of potential. In most cases, he'll work the situation to pulp, as the last thing he wants to do is change.

In the face of inevitable doom, though, his tune will change and his main concern will be to avoid being the bad guy. In his aim for absolution, Taurus will do what he can to get dumped. For him, it's easier to make you do the dirty work than to just fess up. Remember, he's not known to be articulate, and when it comes to emotions, he'll turn into a deaf mute. Usually, he'll start the breakup by dropping subtle hints. Work is his god and the first place he hides when life gets tough. If you're still hanging around while he unapologetically slaves away, he'll make sure he's grumpy when giving you time and then move his asshole-meter up another level. On this level, he'll get forgetful and resilient to commands, which will be his ultimate hint.

In the face of love lost, Taurus gets lazy (and note, there's a difference between comfortable and lazy). He'll do things like have dinner without you, not want to watch your TV shows, sleep the night without spooning you, and/or be uppity about taking out your garbage. He'll test the limits of how far he can go on acting out like a spoiled brat, letting you draw the line. In some awful cases, Taurus will be so dumbfounded with how to deal that he may even take to grunting when communicating with you. It's with these little messages he's asking to be dumped. Best to take your cue, save your energy for a brighter day, and leave to him to his guilt.

. . . And Other Signs He Hates You

When Taurus turns on you, expect to go from red carpet to shit list. He'll hate by getting stingy and refusing to serve. Expect to lug your own shit, deal with disgusting dinners and obligatory sex that'll make you feel like meat. It's a cold place for sure, as he's delivering you back to mortal status. To push the knife in deeper, he'll emphasize his disdain by going out of his way for others in front of your face and disregarding your needs completely. In fact, if you need something, he'll make himself aware of that need and then perform that task for someone else—like your worst enemy.

His inability to say how he feels makes for situations where he acts passive and you get aggressive. You'll want to smack him and jab back with nasty insults, but he'll then make himself the victim while you go mad. He has a smooth way of making you look the fool, as his usually polite demeanor makes people incredulous to his mean streak. Sure, you can push the point, but then you'd have to deal with all his stockpiled rage. If you're brave enough to go there, be prepared to kiss him good-bye once and for all, because once he unravels, there's rarely a way to put him back.

Beating Him to the Punch

The time spent with your Taurus will be the ruler in which he measures your commitment. The less time means the easier the break, as fewer routines have become intertwined. In most cases, he'll be reasonable and want to do what's practical. However, if he's a love-starved Taurus that sticks to you like glue, prepare for a long road ahead.

Getting rid of Taurus effectively takes time, like a termite problem. The one plus is that if you're evil, you can have lots of fun. He's a doormat for love and can spend forever and a day being bossed around, so eradicating him from your life means being able to use him up and wear him thin. Sure, he'll understand you want out if you tell him, but unless you show him by actions that you mean it, he won't truly get it. Like, when you want sex, but don't want to do much work. Go ahead and be the bottom. Need someone to pick up your dry cleaning and then recaulk your tub? Hmm, guess who to call? Yes, drive him to hate you.

Taurus' understanding is that if he works hard at anything, he'll succeed. That's great if you were Lady Liberty, but you're not—so if he just won't go away, make him work for his escape. See, in his demented little mind, he believes that one day you can love him the way he loves you. Logically, we all know this situation can't be easily turned around, and once you treat someone like a slave, they usually don't wind up making you the love of their life—but no one informed Taurus of this. The fact is, he loves love and sometimes that's all he sees. By using him up, he'll hopefully learn there's more to love than doing the dishes or handing over the remote control easily. Whatever the case, it won't be your problem and if you do start to miss him, just hire a butler.

Ridding Yourself of Taurus with Minimal Scarring:

- ♡ Ask for an open relationship. Taurus is typically a serial monogamist.
- ♡ Overwork him thanklessly. He'll crack eventually.
- ♡ Refuse to deal with his family. He'll take it personally and will always choose them over you.

♡ Throw loud parties and leave behind messes. Be wasteful with food while you're at it.

♡ Keep him from sleep by waking him up frequently with silly questions or demands.

♡ Have a super-social schedule that keeps you out all day and night—wanting him to be your arm candy. Be wasteful with money for added effect.

♡ Get him to start an insane fitness routine with you, complete with a totally strict diet.

Kick, Drop, and Kill

Once you feel as if you have no fight left, know you're free and clear to start recovering from running with your bull. Taurus gives up when you give out. However, this is only the beginning to your road to recovery—which tends to be short, because after he's gone you'll notice how many chores have piled up, waiting for your attention. Yes, true heartbreak comes when it's back to domestic duty for you. With the room service gone, you'll get weepy—as that's how Taurus gets you. He spoils you with the little things, and only after the debacle is done will you really understand the depth of affection he tried to express. You might rethink the situation and wonder what's wrong with you; how you could let such a seemingly great guy slip through—but remind yourself: it's the guy on paper, the one who is only palpable in the second dimension, that you'll be mourning. Best to pack away the memories early on and get right to your laundry, taking comfort in learning that there's more to love than just having someone deliver Twinkies and blow jobs to your door.

WANTED: GEMINI

BORN: MAY 23-JUNE 20

Sharply dressed man-child with ambiguous sexual tendencies loaded with charisma and commitment issues. Twitches with a nervous energy and appears when gossip is spoken.

BARE BASICS

How to Spot Him

If you like to talk, laugh incessantly, explore bizarre interests, look stylish and prefer a man who's seemingly cute over intense, then be on the lookout for a youthful character of medium to small stature, slender, dressed in a smart trendy fashion, with a playful twinkle in his eyes, and who chatters on with an inquisitive, yet slightly anxious energy, to anyone in proximity. He's easy to spot and easier to love, as he's too adorable to ignore and has a sense of humor that's harder to resist. To lure him in, be ready with a treasure trove of magic tricks and a pocketful of candy, as that and a little ingenuity is what you'll need to taste the sweet that's known as Gemini.

Always open to new experiences, Gemini is led by his curiosities. In a constant effort to keep his mind stimulated, his biggest fear is boredom. However, how he defines tedium is highly conceptual, as he's a neurotic who can dissect the most innocent occurrences into the worst-case scenarios—but as long as his mind has something to dig deep into, it's okay. To keep his brain from exploding with these

paranoia overloads, Gemini will have at least two different personalities in which to organize all of his thoughts, insanities, interests,
moods, ideologies, etc. On good days, hanging with him feels like
a party. On bad days, it'll feel like being stuck in gridlock traffic with
a thousand horns blaring in your ear.

In highly social areas, chances are higher he'll be on his best
behavior. The more festive, the better, Gemini thrives on large doses
of energy. He's in his element when circulating amid a colorful
mélange of boisterous personalities, being in mid-conversation with
everyone. Multitasking is his thing, and if he can, he'll also be found
dancing and/or being the self-deprecating jokester who keeps the
laughter rolling. If you catch his eye, Gemini's immediate reaction is
to gawk in a state of paralysis or have an irrepressible desire that
bounces him right over, to impress with his clever humor. His talent:
instant endearment. From there, he'll dazzle you with as much can-
did and curious conversation necessary to unleash the chemistry.

In playing up his lovable winsome self, Gemini carries out a
cocky cool with an adorable awkwardness and wraps it in a boyish
package that brings out the youthful energy in anyone he wishes to
possess. It's a power that'll make you want to rip his clothes off and
hump him like a horny teenager (at least for anyone who isn't taller
than him), as he loves to be loved like a pop star. Despite the raven-
ous passion he stirs, though, the ambiance he casts is light and
tinged with a harmless and delicious flirtation. Gemini's goal: create
a puppy-love world to get lost in and source out a paradise for his
non-threatening ass to bury his bone—his usually very lively and
pretty bone, that is. Just give him the word and make him fetch.

Key Features:

- A small stature, usually, in body frame and height
- A bigger head size than normal
- Twinkly excitable eyes set in a boyish face

- ♡ A youthful style, somewhat of a fashion victim
- ♡ Looks as if his sexuality is debatable
- ♡ Good with words, a great sense of humor, Curious and inquisitive—expect him to ask lots of questions straight off
- ♡ Found in social environments that are trendy and busy— usually talking

Seducing Him into Your Boudoir

Flirting is second nature to Gemini. He's so playful; not even he'll know when he's being for real or just teasing. If the urge hits, it hits. If not, oh well. To say the least, this guy's not much of a planner and it's not so much that he's moody, as much as it's that he's incredibly indecisive—but that's him and it's the way he likes it. It gives him a rush to teeter on a cliffhanger, even if it's by his own devices. Gemini loves choices, so if you're determined to taste the fruit of his loins, you better be steadfast in your quest and know how to cut his duality off at the pass.

The surefire way to rope in Gemini is with sheer wit. He's got such a mercurial way about him and can entertain himself for hours, looping his mind in circles with the most peculiar topics. To pull him from that and get him to focus on you is the challenge. It'll require nothing less than a personality that pops, chokeholds his attention, and melts his mind with endless fascinations. Mystify him with your smart, sexy, and comedic ways and overwhelm his brain to think of nothing but you. Ooze from every pore with a fearless charm and give him a run for his money. Move fast and think even faster. Offer up interesting banter, filled with strange trivia and tons more humor. Get him to laugh and he'll be putty in your hands. In speeding up Gemini's brainwave, you'll get a rise out of him that you're sure to enjoy.

By showing him you can add to the excitement he already stirs, you'll prove yourself worthy to be his match. Once that mission has been accomplished, he'll make his intentions blaringly apparent, as he's a hands-on kind of guy. However, realize Gemini does have an ADD way about him, making his window of opportunity small. If you don't jump fast, his neurotic energy might get him too drunk or nervous to fuck, as his mojo is never consistent (or anything about him). Best not to take chances. Besides, Gemini's best performances are typically impromptu ones and a memorable adventure not to be missed. He's way more fun than a roller coaster, and coincidentally they both take about the same time for you to get off on as well. So, if you have a few minutes to spare, ride one.

Loving Him in the Boudoir

Don't expect Gemini to give you epic sex that'll last for hours building you up to a giant crescendo climax; accept that fact now and you won't be disappointed. As the master of the quickie, Gemini sex is more about getting off swiftly, vigorously, and interestingly. Not known for longevity with anything he does, what Gemini lacks in longevity he makes up for with surprise and enthusiasm. Being that he needs a thousand things going on at once to keep his mind at peak levels, this carries over rather nicely in the boudoir. While others give sex that's hearty and filling like a steak dinner, Gemini's sex is more like a tapas bar—lots of exciting little tasty treats that satisfy through variety.

With Gemini you never get straight screwing, that would bore him to tears. With him, it's about creating a fun and exciting experience, exploring as much as possible. Sex is a whole bag of tricks, not just one plain fuck. Anything that tickles his curiosity, he'll throw it in and want you to be as open, too. Sex toys, bring it on. More people, sure, why not? The opposite sex, the same sex—what the hell! Out in public or dressed up in costume, okay. You only live once and he's out to try it all. Nothing scares him, and if it does, he'll eventually want to do it.

Plus, being that Gemini is so youthful he fucks as spirited as a teenager. However, his motor skills are all man. Being the ruler of the hands, he has the dexterity of a consummate lover in his. Whatever he touches, he leaves in sheer bliss, as he integrates imagination into all his movements and loves to source out all your sensitive spots that can't resist pleasure. Also, let's not forget he loves to talk, so expect dirty words to spill from his mouth when unoccupied. (If it's not your thing, you can also tell him to "Shut up"; that'll turn him on, too.) All the while, the mood he'll create will be jovial and casual, to avoid any performance anxiety. It's a talent that allows him to be a total slut, as he's perfected pulling off festively kinky exchanges that charge the mind and body, but keep emotions at bay. Not to say he's not capable of that, but generally that's not his forte. Of course, if you keep expanding the scope of his curiosities and playing out fantasies, it's "never say never" for him.

MAKING HIM COME TO THE PALM OF YOUR HAND

Eye Candy

Make no mistake about his depth, despite his ability to hold riveting ten-minute conversations, Gemini is as superficial and judgmental as they get. If you want to last, look good. Image is a priority. Score points by working a style that says young, funky, free, fun, and absurdly fashionable. If not, he'll wonder if you have any sense of humor—and that'll automatically put you on the wrong foot. With Gemini, fashion is an expression, a way to show you're better than everyone else. If you can bond on this level with him, then consider yourself halfway to being in love. Dress with no joie de vivre and count the hours until he dumps you.

Stylin' Seduction:

- ♡ Color. No grim washout looks in all black or gray. Think flamboyance and then go up another notch. Colors that grab him will be electric blue and silver.
- ♡ Trendy styles. He's a fashion victim through and through.
- ♡ Youthful outfits. Clothes that exude a playful and energetic spirit will appeal to him.
- ♡ Androgynous to cross-dressing influences. He loves sexuality as a style.
- ♡ Casual and sporty clothes. Don't worry. He doesn't dig this look because he loves athletic types, but because it's chic to look active.
- ♡ Accessories are a must. Clothes are a palate; accessories are the life of a look.
- ♡ Good hair. He likes his lover styled from head to toe.

Tasty Treats

Food

Gemini would rather talk than chew, making him a finicky eater. Food needs to be a quick shot of deliciousness to render his mouth quiet. Never do long and drawn-out dining experiences, unless there's tons of variety and finger food action. Plus, another prerequisite to dining success is speedy service. Patience is not his virtue and indecisiveness is his craft. He'll scan a menu and needs to get what he wants fast. Otherwise, a flip in choice can occur, and before you know it, he'll obsess over what he can't have. This then blows his whole mood. Yeah, with him, it's like feeding a five-year-old. Give him something quick that he can pick at, play with, and remain non-committal to and he's happier than a pig in shit.

Erotic Eats:

- ♡ Tapas. Variety is the spice of his life.
- ♡ Sushi. It's light and colorful—plus, he can choose from a selection.
- ♡ Cafes with lots of desserts. Gemini loves sugar.
- ♡ Any smorgasbord or buffet where he can mix and match. The more kitsch the better.
- ♡ A trendy restaurant that's cool to be seen in and good for spotting important people. He loves to be in a place where he can gossip about the people.
- ♡ Ethiopian food, medieval times, or any place with a big appetizer menu filled with finger foods. Any place he can eat with his hands will be a hit with him.
- ♡ A supper club. His thinking: The more activities under one roof, the better the food will taste.

Movies

Gemini is either in high-speed motion or zoned out; this is a major thing to know when taking him to the cineplex. While most get fidgety if you make them sit anywhere for long durations, a movie is where you'll have the best chance of getting him to chill. However, you'll need a well-paced plot with action, tension, cinematography, beautiful and poignant dialogue, and preferably a hot cast. He must also be bombarded with constant enthrallment via comedy, drama, or thought-provoking intrigue. In other words, keep Gemini's curiosity perpetually piqued with cinema that can fling his emotions around like a hot potato and twist his mind into a pretzel. Anything less would drain the living shit out of him.

Cinematic Foreplay:

- ♡ Comedies. Base the types on how high- or lowbrow your Gemini's mood is. Slapstick for the more kind-hearted lovable one or black comedy for the intellectual twin.
- ♡ Geeky teen movies. All Geminis have an attachment to their formative years.
- ♡ Indies. He likes to be "in."
- ♡ Psychological thrillers. He loves a good mental tease.
- ♡ B-movies. He can never have enough camp.
- ♡ Short films. He has a short attention span, so these have a better chance of keeping his interest. If they have a unifying theme, even better.
- ♡ Disaster movies. This will appeal to his Mr. Hyde side.

Dating Ideas

Play it by ear and spring plans the day you get together with a few selections that Gemini can mix and match. Automatically, you're percolating his mind and body, as he loves surprises and choices. Anything that promotes conversation, put on the voting ballot, as his main love is to talk; best to give him something you can both discuss. As for the places and pursuits where he'll thrive, go where it's lively, as in plenty of sights and sounds that ideally he can interact with and let his curiosity go wild on. He's an inquisitive creature who thrives when there's plenty of territory he can run his mind and little legs around in.

Playful Planning:

- ♡ A planetarium or science museum. He thrives in places with lots of things to touch and snippets of trivia to learn.
- ♡ A picnic in a scenic environment to talk, people-watch, or play a board game. If he's somewhere with lots to look at, the better the chance of him staying in one spot.

♡ Mini-golf, go-karts, or any other interactive low-impact sport. He needs to be on the move, but it can't be demanding.

♡ A party. He loves meeting new people and chatting them up.

♡ A comedy club. He thinks himself a comedian.

♡ A short day trip anywhere. Gemini loves brief adventures.

♡ A nightclub. He's got tons of energy to burn, and most playful Geminis love tripping the light fantastic—even if most do dance as if they're on drugs.

Sound Seduction

Conversation

Everything is open for discussion. From the absolutely absurd to the painfully poignant, the more variety the better, as Gemini just loves questioning and answering anything, creating more to think and talk about. As ruled by Mercury, Gemini loves communicating. The more tangents you provide, the more he'll be engaged. However, it's not that he likes talking about himself or anything personal, unless it's gossip or trivia. It's about flexing his mind and mouth in as many extremes as possible, from hardcore problem solving to irrelevant mumble jumble and anything in between. Have plenty of subjects to bounce around to create a conversational necklace and he'll pleasantly link it together with his lively flow of non sequiturs.

Icebreakers:

♡ Find out who are the five people he'd have for a sleepover, alive or dead, and why. Fantasy hypothetical questions are his favorite.

♡ Ask whether he would rather drink a half-gallon of liquid trash from a mall's food court or have to suck on a homeless man's big toe for thirty minutes. He's always keen on "would you rather" questions. He loves pondering impossible situations.

♡ Ask him about when he was a teen. Geminis love reminiscing about their formative years.

♡ If he were stranded on an island for a year, what ten things would he bring? All the essentials are already there, like clothes, but not his. He loves questions with details.

♡ Ask about his most embarrassing moments. He'll have hours of funny stories.

♡ If he could have one superhero power, what would it be? What would he do with it? Multi-prong questions and answers with different layers are always tops with him.

♡ Ask him brainteasers, such as: What English word can have four of its five letters removed and still retains its original pronunciation? (*Answer: Queue.*) Brainteasers are his idea of fun.

Music

Silence isn't Gemini's thing. With a brain that swings from obsessive neurotic to happy freak erratically and frequently, music helps his mind focus. It gives him something to anchor his mood and drown out the voices in his head. Any kind of busy-sounding music that's uplifting is his taste and preferably with lyrical prose that'll move his mind. If the beat can make him shake his booty, too, even better. (Unless he's the old-man Gemini who is too self-conscious to deal.) Being that he's like a transmitter, first his mind will tune in and then his body.

Mood Makers:

♡ Disco/dance music. He loves to groove.

♡ Klezmer. He's just that unique!

♡ Funk/psychedelic. Anything that'll make him move works with him.

♡ Dixieland. Its energy exemplifies Gemini.

♡ Pop music, as long as it's smart. Japanese pop—even better, as it's hyper-fast and cute.

♡ Alternative. Whatever is current will appeal to his trendy side.
♡ Songs with well-written lyrics. He's got a literary thing going on and words are important to him.

Gifts

Doing anything with his hands excites him, but none as intoxicating as unwrapping a present. Gemini loves gifts and especially when it's a surprise. This means getting presents for no reason is more his speed than for holidays or birthdays. For Gemini, it's more about being showered with little mementos that spontaneously inspire you to think of him that'll touch him. The good news is you don't have to break the bank to please him. The bad news is you better be imaginative when it comes to nailing items that'll reflect his finicky personality and frequently present these morsels of love to him.

Boxed Treats:

♡ Notebooks. Geminis love to write, even if it's just the physical act of doing it.
♡ Magazine subscriptions or books. Gemini rules media and these are the types of gifts that keep giving.
♡ Small gadgets. Anything he can play with and carry around, as he's a fidgeter.
♡ Practical joke gifts. He's the original jokester of the zodiac.
♡ Camera-related presents. Photography is in Gemini's blood.
♡ Clothes or accessories. He can't resist fashion.
♡ Video games. It's something for his hands and mind—perfect.

Touch Me

Gemini wants sex like fingerprints: to never have the same experience twice. As a man who equates boredom to a terminal illness, to do him good means having endless tricks up your sleeve and the ability to juggle them out fast, formidably, and flexibly. He gets off on enthusiasm, energy, and the element of surprise. The more you can catch him off guard with new thrills and sensations, the stronger his drive gets. In reality, Gemini isn't the most sexually needy creature and it takes effort to heat him up. While he has no problem being a big ole flirt who loves attention, it isn't necessarily because of his libido or ego, but more of a social skill. What really does grab his attention and makes him hard is when you work his most important muscle: his brain.

Being that he's an ADD kind of guy, it's not that Gemini likes it kinky, he needs it so. To have any worthwhile sex with him means offering a twist. To get him hard, he needs to be fascinated with an endless wonderland of mental and physical delights. Sex with Gemini is best when it's spontaneous, playful, and sweet. He prefers a causal approach, with a lover who can challenge his mind and body. So share your savvy wit and live out sexual experiences that can integrate as much variety as possible. Toys, games, extra people, peculiar places, dirty talk, or any added element that heightens his mental stimulus works, as it'll give him more to think about and, most important, more to talk about.

Of course, how you incorporate these added accoutrements to create your dirty little trysts must also be considered. Know that if you pack the most into a short span of time, the better he'll be. Anything, even freaky sex, with a long time frame isn't fun for Gemini. Break it up with scintillating conversation between sets and costume changes and/or move to various locations, always keeping it fresh. Just be sure you don't spoil him too much and spring the sexcapades on him in random doses. It's all about keeping your sex as a novelty—that'll help keep him titillated and inquisitive in and out of the boudoir, as ultimately curiosity is Gemini's aphrodisiac.

Ways to Heat Up Your Gemini:

- ♡ Massage his hands in a sexual kind of way, that's where you can find his erogenous zone.
- ♡ Send him dirty letters and pictures through e mail or cell phone—any racy communication will appease the pervert in him.
- ♡ Be spontaneous; take him in various places and keep switch-ing up the styles.
- ♡ Do him in a car or any form of transportation; multitask the sex, he's all for it.
- ♡ Use costumes and play games. The element of surprise goes a long way with him.
- ♡ Be his secret admirer and send him several weeks or months of letters describing your attraction to him and the things you want to do to him, but don't reveal your identity quickly. Tease him and then spring it on him.
- ♡ Invite newcomers. He's the most likely of the zodiac to want to swing.

Role-playing

Geminis make great actors. Each are born with a closet full of per-sonalities that they'll dive into periodically. Just request a character or wait ten minutes and you'll see how versatile he is. For Gemini, life is too complicated to just be one person, not to mention too dull. His reasoning: Why see the world from one point of view when you can see it through a thousand? Obviously, with this philosophy he's a natural-born role-player. While he'll be open to anything, he'll get off better with interaction between opposites and a focus on dia-logue. Also, the scenes he'll get into are those where he can relive past events in his life, recreating it the way he wanted them in the first place. Editing is an inherent skill; so perfecting his memories is another resource of endless Gemini indulgence.

Cast of Characters:

- ♡ Each other. You play him and he can be you. It's a psychological challenge that'll be an additional boost in getting him off.
- ♡ Astronaut and alien. Make love on the alien's planet. The outer space theme will appeal to him.
- ♡ Geeky teens on prom night for the first time. All Geminis have nostalgia for their teen years.
- ♡ Your favorite romantic movie parts. Geminis are great actors.
- ♡ Porn stars making porn for foreign TV. It's raunchy, but with a twist—perfect for him to flex his imagination!
- ♡ Each chooses a random person. Make sure it is someone you both know, and do it as that mystery person. The object of this game is to figure out who you're fucking. He loves games!
- ♡ Online daters that have been having virtual sex with each other, then decide to get it on in person. Yes, start this one on a computer, then work your way into the bedroom. This will allow him to use his brain first, body second—the way he likes it.

Taking the Bait

Gemini loves love and its giddy obsession that drives him right into fairy tale mode—where he loves to get lost and live out his Peter Pan fantasies. He works non-stop, too, to perpetuate this dreamy world, making you feel like the most precious creature to ever grace his world by wooing you with witty surprises, sweet words, and endless comic relief. With such magic in the air when you two connect, it'd be impossible to think he's not as head-over-heels as you are. After all, who could resist the boundless fun, sidesplitting laugh-a-minute moments, and conversations that last past sunrise? It would seem surreal to think you're not a match made in heaven. So, silly you, you mention the future or something vague that acknowledges your bond . . .

Little does anyone know what brews in this man's mind, least of all Gemini.

Welcome to the dark side of Gemini. You heard the warnings, perhaps read the books. Yes, this guy can flip at the drop of a hat. Despite being in a state of bliss, his mind is set on an automatic timer that goes off when any remote hint of responsibility comes into play. Then, out goes his Dr. Jekyll and in comes his Mr. Hyde, ready to scrutinize and freak out.

Being that Gemini loves having millions of possibilities, when faced with any crossroads of change, he'll schitz. It won't matter how chill you are or how happy your relationship is, he'll see it as a possible doom—doom of his freedom and identity. With so many voices in his head, he'll wonder if he can handle yet another one that's outside of him—that voice being you. When he is faced with the side of love that isn't just about fantasy sex and perfect days, it forces him to deal with his priorities. To figure out what they are, he shuts down to search for an epiphany. If he's MIA twenty-four hours or less, it's normal. If not, it's a red flag.

Upon resurfacing, it'll be Gemini #1, but acting as if he's just returned from an abduction. At that moment, he'll take responsibilities for his actions and articulate all his innermost feelings, thought processes, and tips with how to deal with him. Basically, he'll give you the key that opens himself to you. While it's not the most sooth-ing method, it can explain why he worked so hard in the beginning, hoping to compensate for the jackass he knew would spring out of him eventually. It sucks, but yeah, only when you meet his Mr. Hyde and his humbled Dr. Jekyll will you truly know his truth, making it up to you to love them or leave them.

UNAUTHORIZED: ASTRAL AUTOPSY

Recognizing Fear

Boredom is death to Gemini. Without anything to sufficiently occupy his brain, he's a goner. If this means being a neurotic, living to worry, so be it. At least that gives himself something he can always do. Even though it sounds like a torturous state to subject oneself to, it does put his chronic state of ennui into remission—which he considers the worst torture, because it might make him think it's really him that's boring and not the world around him.

Main cause
Being or feeling dull.

Immunizing His Fears:

- ♡ Have a variety of topics and keep the conversation rolling. Silence is deadly.
- ♡ When he starts to feel nervous, which will be obvious by his inability to focus his eyes, ask a lot of questions. It may confuse him, but confusion easily trumps fear.
- ♡ Return his calls quickly and confirm plans every two seconds. Keep the communication fast and constant.
- ♡ Keep him laughing. Light atmospheres ease his mind.
- ♡ Medicate him. Pills, booze, whatever you've got. He loves chemicals! Not PC, but 100 percent effective.

Infecting Him with Fear:

- ♡ Suggest he's boring, which is his biggest fear.
- ♡ Tell him to turn off his cell phone when he's with you. This will make him feel as if he's cut off from the universe and fearfully isolated.

♥ Suggest he's old, like laugh at his music tastes for being outdated or tell him his shoes are so last season. He's all about
his youthfulness. Dorian Gray was most likely a Gemini.

♡ Tell everyone a secret, but him. He's an information hound;
without it, he goes insane.

♡ Stick to him like glue. He's a claustrophobic type and needs
lots of space, physically and mentally.

Recognizing Anger

In general, Gemini guards against feeling angry. Getting mad is a
buzz kill and he hates being brought down (unless he's alone, but
that's another story you'll read about shortly . . .). He keeps a jovial
attitude, as he likes conversations not arguments. Of course, there
are going to be those moments when life speeds up and words
escape him. When left speechless or unable to express himself, he
responds with agitation. At those moments his anger will seep out,
resembling that of a frustrated baby.

Main cause
An inability to communicate his thoughts and emotions articulately.

Immunizing His Anger:

♡ Make a clever joke about his fury. He has a short attention
span for everything, and charming him out of anger is quite
easy in most cases.

♡ Give him a hand massage. His anger can easily get shifted
with physical pleasure.

♡ Whatever he's mad at, let him go on about it. Soon enough,
he'll change subjects himself, as staying on one isn't his style.

♡ Give him candy and/or tickle him. The same things that
would work at quelling a toddler usually work on Gemini
too.

♡ Diffuse his anger by changing the focus to your anger. He'll shift into a defense mode automatically. He easily flows where the conversation flows.

Infecting Him with Anger:

♡ Cut him off whenever he speaks. The frustration will make him explode.

♡ Yawn at his opinions and call him out when he misquotes facts. He thinks of himself as a purveyor of information. Ruin his illusion; deal with his wrath.

♡ Don't laugh at his jokes. He prides himself on his humor. Instead of thinking he's not funny, he'll blame you for not getting it.

♡ Ruin his shots when he's taking a picture. Geminis have a thing for photography and they're all serious about their "art." If you're in a car and he's trying to shoot something, speed up so he misses it—things like this will infuriate him indefinitely.

♡ Read his newspaper or magazine before him and leak the info before he reads it.

Recognizing Sadness

You'd never suspect it by looking at him, but Gemini has a dark side that can suck the life out of you. It's his "not so secret" dirty little secret, and in the lonely hours of his existence, it comes out via his evil twin who flogs his ego to a pulp and undermines any shred of happiness he has mustered for himself. This is his sadness and what he feels gives him depth. Yes, for every laugh he belts out is a tear that'll pour out in his solitude. This is one of the main reasons why so many Geminis tend to be so social. By transforming himself into a performer, he can hide behind others and use the audience's acceptance as his calming elixir. Sure, sometimes it helps if he can be tuned out pharmaceutically, too, as it's just about getting himself through the day.

Main cause
With a brain that travels at the speed of light, it's inevitable he'll hit a few bumps along the way.

Immunizing His Sadness:

♡ Gossip. Nothing like talking about other people's messed-up lives to derail his own tragedies.

♡ Load him up with books on the subject of his misery. Collecting info always keeps him content.

♡ Take him shopping. It's the perfect outlet for his compulsions.

♡ Respond quickly to his communications and with long responses. This includes regular mail, e-mail, texts, picture messages, etc.

♡ Take him out. Being social cures all, as he'll have to turn on his charm.

Infecting Him with Sorrow:

♡ Ignore his comments or misquote him when talking to others and have him overhear.

♡ When out with him, tell him your tired. If you're not as energetic as him 24-7, he'll take it personally.

♡ Go out, have tons of fun, and then split suddenly. By pumping him up with happiness, being alone will deflate him soon enough.

♡ Use big words he won't know. He has a phobia about his intelligence. Prey on it.

♡ Create a routine and break his spirit by regimenting him.

Recognizing Trust

Trust is a form of commitment, a subject he'd rather avoid. Gemini is way too changeable to rely on even his own thoughts, let alone anyone else's. With trust, it's given out like a day pass to an amusement park—good for a taste of the fun and excitement and taken back when he's too pooped to be nice. Ultimately, trust requires too much responsibility and he'd prefer submitting only when necessary, as he's fine with the flexibility to be a smidgen flakey. The way around all it is to assume his trust and never question it, because once it gets examined is when he'll feel trapped.

Main cause
It's something you got to give to get.

Immunizing with Trust:

♡ Ask his advice and take it more than once. If you trust him, he can trust you.

♡ Have a high IQ and prove it, like showing off high SAT scores. Intelligence equals trustworthiness.

♡ Have lots of magazine subscriptions, know websites, and own tons of books. Looking informed will have him believe you are.

♡ Reveal your dark side. Only when he sees you're schized like him can he understand you better. The more he can understand you, the more he can trust you.

♡ If you have good taste or are attractive, he'll be more prone to want to trust you. He's superficial. Enough said.

Infecting His Trust:

♡ Create neurosis through communication. Tell him you hang up on people on purpose when you're on the cell and blame it on a bad connection. Then shortly after, get "cut off" with him.

♡ Gossip or flirt as much as he does. Nothing like giving him a dose of his own medicine to make him feel like he's on shaky ground.

♡ Be a bad listener a few times and it'll mar your record permanently. Have him catch you zoning out while talking to him.

♡ Need to read directions word for word. He doesn't trust people who play by the rules or has the attention span to know them.

♡ Ignore your gut reactions. If you don't listen to them, he'll be suspicious about how you do form your decisions.

Recognizing Motivation

Keeping active is never the issue with Gemini; being focused is his Achilles' heel. While he'll go anywhere the mood strikes and travel to the ends of earth to quell his curiosities, it needs to be on his terms. He's a commitmentphobe, so moving him along must be done by suggestion. Talk around a subject and get him to ask questions. His inquisitiveness is his fuel. Of course, whatever the subject, it must be fun, mind-expanding, and interactive. Without those three elements, he'll have no interest.

Main cause
Curiosity keeps his ass moving.

Immunizing His Motivation:

♡ Involve him in any long-term projects. Like his typical stature size, he needs things short.

♡ Confuse him with many details and questions. When given too much info, he'll generally detour from the main focus.

♡ Have rules. He hates them. Things need to be flexible, as that's the one thing about him that won't bend.

♡ Make things repetitious; he'll eventually fall asleep. He operates best with multifaceted situations.

♡ Use dry words; this will bore him and make his interest fade on any subject you discuss.

Infecting Him with Motivation:

♡ Make a game out of everything. He thrives with playful settings.

♡ If he hears something is cool, he'll want to check it out. Image is everything to Gemini.

♡ Create dialogues to spur his curiosity. Talk gives his interest something to hold on to.

♡ Leave little slips of paper lying about so Gemini will read them. If you want to get him interested in going somewhere you want, leave a magazine open to an article about it or pamphlets on the matter. It'll be the only suggestion you'll need to give, to get him to want to find out more.

♡ Give him a task and pose it as a test to prove his intelligence, and he'll get focused fast.

DESTINATION: DUMPSVILLE

Celestial Voodoo on You

Gemini's multiple personalities make him hard to read and trust. He'll be your biggest fan one minute, then treat you like a contagious spore the next. It's nothing personal, either, but his dark side is a contentious child who will act out periodically. Who the hell this fucker really is can be difficult to pinpoint and possibly a nightmare to try to have a relationship with—as there are too many in him to deal. The worst part is there's no one you can ask, because he won't even know why he feels the way he does. To him, it's normal. So, with this said, find a good psychic if you want a clue about the end, because just like Armageddon it can be sudden and unprovoked.

Once Gemini starts to feel vaguely bored, trapped, or anything negative, his first instinct is to bolt. Sure he needs to have his space to think, but when it comes to the end, it means that his dark side will come out to be his rep and there'll be no talking any logic with him. In submitting himself to another, he has a fear of losing his identity—or in his case, identities. Being caught in thinking "we, not just me" leaves him feeling claustrophobic and responsible for too many people. Gemini's solution? Make one decision—go. Then, when it comes to revealing his revelation, he'll have the gracefulness of a giraffe on roller skates.

In the face of being serious or trying to sound sincere with his emotions, he'll get inarticulate and quiet. Fumbling with words, Gemini avoids wanting to be hurtful, yet he has no ability to sound nurturing. Inevitably, he'll be wishy-washy. In seeing this side, it makes it quite clear who he is and what he's all about. Of course, if you play nice and sympathetic to his pathetic state, this can be to your detriment, as it'll open him up back into being indecisive. If this is the case, he'll act like a chronic disease that pulls you back to worship you, then acts unruly, then pledges his undying love again, and then wants to dump you again. If you give him the power to have his cake and eat it too, then he'll take it all the way, which is why it's important for someone to be the adult and put a stop to Gemini's vicious cycles.

. . . And Other Signs He Hates You

When Gemini deems you an enemy, expect to hear all about it. Immediately, in hating you, he'll take on a superior and condescending attitude. Gone is the funny man with the jovial expression, and in comes his drill sergeant who speaks in as few syllables as needed and in as somber a manner as possible. Then, behind your back he'll talk crap, passing all the gossip he has on you. Yes, his approach is typically very high school playground, trying to gain the popular vote any way he can. When it gets down to it, though, this ploy works out great because he can filter out the losers you really don't want to know—mostly him. Obviously, not responding back is the way to deflect his immaturity, but because he's so silly with his rancid tongue, it's even better to laugh back in his face when he attempts to spit out his fire.

Beating Him to the Punch

Want to make Gemini love you more? Dump him. He's a sufferer of the grass-is-greener syndrome, and whenever you tell him, "No," all he'll want to do is get you to say, "Yes." He's an irrepressible brat who, when caught in this trifling situation, will typically respond with doing what he loves best—talk and in details, over and over again. He'll have a list of questions three miles long and go on even longer pointless diatribes that won't do anything, but aggravate you more. To avoid this travesty, make the breakup brief: Approach stoically, say what you must, and leave. If possible, pencil him in between appointments so you have no time to listen to anything, but his "bye." After, ignore all contact; block if possible. Don't respond to his calls, e-mail, IM, text messages, or anything else. Erase before opening or listening, as it might tempt you. For Gemini, silencing him is the worst torture possible. Soon enough, refusing him his communication will drive him to a conniption, but as long as it's not in your presence, will it matter? If a tree falls in the forest, does it make a sound? A dumped Gemini soon finds out that answer.

Ridding Yourself of Gemini with Minimal Scarring:

♡ Need him emotionally. That's sure to freak him out completely.
♡ Take several days to call him back. That'll bug him to no end.

♡ Half-heartedly listen to him and put words in his mouth.
♡ Be boring or worse: Tell him he's boring.
♡ Be slow with everything, talking, walking, thinking, etc.
♡ Nag him and be no fun. He hates condescension, unless he's doling it out.
♡ Be insatiable. He loves sex, but at most once a day. If you demand too much, he'll snap soon enough.

Kick, Drop, and Kill

Gemini starts off with so much promise, but as soon as he starts going on too much and off on too many tangents it's quite obvious he's got his own thing going on. Everyone else is just his sidekick sounding board who can enjoy his entertainment or not, as he's not changing for anyone. If anyone dares to try to make him change, he'll then unveil his bully, via his dark side. From there it can be any-one's guess who or what will unravel. Walking away from him is much like eradicating a boil from your ass; it may take some patience to get him through your system, but as the clarity returns, so does your confidence.

The nice thing about Gemini, though, is that he's fun and has a talent to bring about a carefree feeling, like visiting a fairy wonder-land where anything can happen. Unfortunately, it couldn't always be that way, as consistency isn't his strong suit. So, as he flutters back into Never Neverland, you can be grateful for one thing: his ability to show you the key to that magic world and why you love it there. While it might never be him that enters in with you, there'll always be that glimmer of hope, a curiosity that'll burn in your mind that perhaps one day he can balance himself out to be a boyish man rather than a mannish boy. Yeah, it can keep you guessing, but that's him, always leaving something behind to think about.

WANTED: CANCER

BORN: JUNE 21–JULY 22

Seductive sourpuss with a tendency to camouflage himself into the background. Likes to assume invisibility and then sulk about no one noticing him. Has a signature pout and lures you in to ignore you.

BARE BASICS

How to Spot Him

Break out the telescope if you want to spot a Cancer. More elusive than Haley's Comet, this domestic homebody doesn't make it a regular thing to mix and mingle out in society. If he does, he prefers to slink around alone in the outskirts of a crowd and blend in with the furniture. You might encounter him if you accidentally sit on him or have to move around him to get to the bathroom. If he says nothing, it's his bad day and best to move on. If he says, "Hi," it's a good day and you should feel free to plant yourself down, because when he's feeling the love there's nothing more soothing than bonding souls with this lovely and most delicate creature.

Yes, Cancer can be a total disaster when it comes to making first impressions. Being that he has the propensity to be the moodiest son of a bitch ever, it's a toss-up with how he'll react. Every aspect of his life is a factor at every moment: who he's with, where he's at, what he's wearing, what's in his bank account, etc. Everything is blended to create his emotional chemistry, which will result in a time bomb of fun or fury. He's a serious man, and nothing is ever taken lightly. It's 110 percent intensity 247, and that means even when he's having fun.

At worst, he turns invisible and then gets upset when no one acknowledges his grumpiness. All the while, he'll have gleam in his eye, scanning the room like a security camera and sizing up every thing in his path. In this mode, Cancer's out to play judgment day—with you in the hot seat. In being the outsider, he'll think he knows all and will state his opinions as fact. Sure, he'll be right 97 percent of the time, but who likes a bitter know-it-all who only sees half the picture?

Of course, with that warning said, understand Cancer's egregious social skills tend to be his defense mechanism to protect his soft, gushy, and sensitive side that lies beneath. To ensure his safety, he'll need to be withdrawn—unless his biorhythms are up and he's loaded with confidence to reveal his kind, nurturing, open side by way of being excessively cheery and flirtatious, darting about to everyone as if he's running for office. He'll have the exuberance of a prisoner set free (aka his self-hating cage), almost to the point of being too over the top and nutty. No, he's not for everyone, but if you're that "one in a thousand" person who can get on his rocky wavelength, he'll be just what you need. Armed with an intuition that can reach into the deepest depths of your soul, he'll be able to comfort your most private parts that you never thought anyone would understand. Sure, he's a walking jack-in-the-box surging with a cornucopia of delights and damnations, but when such a karmic connection is made, destiny makes him irresistible.

Key Features:

- ♡ A defined chest that sticks out when scared or feeling boastful
- ♡ Premature gray hairs/an older face than the age he reveals
- ♡ A round face
- ♡ Tendency to have a belly
- ♡ A blended-in style that makes him undetectable in a crowd

♡ Shy approach to things or completely in your face and over the top

♡ When not withdrawn, can have a smothering energy and gets too close and in your personal space when talking to you

Seducing Him into Your Boudoir

Cancer loves romance and all aspects of courting, except sticking to roles. If anyone is going to get chased, he wants to be the one. It's easier for him to play on the offensive than on the defensive, as he's totally neurotic and overly cautious. You can grow old waiting for him to make a move; best to jump into the driver's seat ASAP. Once in place, rev his motor by opening up yourself pronto. Despite his turtle-like ways, he's looking to bond and feel the love fast. In baring your soul he'll show you his, and together you can cut to the chase. His objective: paint a bigger picture and see where you can fit in his scheme of things. The more you understand him, the more he'll draw you in.

As a man out to commit and be committed, Cancer plays for keeps—and we're talking love that's about you and him against the world. Not one to do anything lightly, he'll immediately need to see your depth, compassion, creativity, and willingness to put up with him. He knows he's not an easy person to love, and to even think of opening himself up will cause him to put up a wall to see how you break through. Not that he's mean about it, per se, but he's out for unconditional love, and to find it he has to be a little abrasive around the edges. Yes, it's a tall order for anyone to fill, especially in the early stages, but it's the game he plays and most probably the reason why he gets so grumpy. Being that he has such lofty standards, it's a big bummer to see that the world won't generally work that way. Of course, Cancer figures in time he's got to hit the jackpot, right? Right. After all, you're reading this.

So, in a nutshell, if you want him, be prepared to dive into the intensity. Don't worry; if you've got what it takes, you'll get back ten times more. Just know you need to nurture the fuck out of him and be able to listen to him endlessly go on about his trials and tribulations. Mother him, but don't baby him. If you can handle his heat/whininess, then consider yourself spoken for. No, it's not the sexiest way to snatch up a man, but this is Cancer and he's way more evolved than having to play hard to get.

Loving Him in the Boudoir

Cancer is all the way in or all the way out. When he's snapped you up, be ready to be possessed like you've never been possessed before. While some may think it feels like being a kidnap victim, others find this sort of romance nice and cozy. Imagine being with someone who loves you like a stalker, but doesn't scare you like one. It's a little maddening, but hell, so is love and this is his style. He lives to make his lovers feel good and completely taken care of. Call it being protective or overly possessive, but when you're in Cancer's world, he's out to rock it 100 percent.

In the boudoir, expect to feel every emotion Cancer has for you. His love is passionate and filled with intensity. He has no limits on the romance he offers and this will include all the traditional precursors to sex—like the wining, dining, flowers, and candy. He's all for the emotional foreplay before getting naked. In bed, he's omnipresent and aiming to make a spiritual bond each time he enters. Hell, half the time it isn't so much the sex that'll get him off, as it's the pre- and post-coitus cuddling. Yeah, he's into the affection big time and gives himself over wholly, but that's just one mood to him. Remember, he has lots of secrets brewing inside him, and just when you think you can pinpoint his style, he'll flip it around.

To every doting and sweet side of Cancer lies a dark side. If he's in a gray phase of his day and feeling frisky, expect him to approach primally and perform sex as if he's marking his territory.

Being so delicate, he hits a wall and then bounces into feeling like he has to be "a man." When he's there, it can be quite exciting, as he's unpredictable. This sex will be aggressive and somewhat rough. While he never mixes the two modes in one session, he'll give you the best of both worlds as he feels it. Sexually, he'll reveal himself a little at a time. So, if you like mystery, you'll love Cancer.

MAKING HIM COME TO THE PALM OF YOUR HAND

Eye Candy

Cancer man is Mr. Au Naturel. He already has so many things to consider about his lovers that the last thing he needs to worry about is their wardrobe. His preference is uncomplicated looks and lovers who are adorned as simply as possible, pure if doable—as in appearance only. What he sees is what he wants to get. This means no heavy makeup, flamboyant clothing, or big teased-out and sprayed-up hair. He's streamlined and finds classic looks that border on prim and proper to be his kind of sexy. There's no need to break the bank to dress for this man either; best to save your money on sex toys instead.

Stylin' Seduction:

- ♡ Natural colors and subtle prints, if any. However, solid-color clothes are more his speed. Colors that turn him on: white and silver.
- ♡ Form-fitted clothes that are sexy, not slutty. Think hemlines suitable for religious occasions.
- ♡ Sporty casual and subtle style, clothes that can make you blend in with a crowd.

♡ Anything that reveals your chest. He is the ruler of that area and just loves it like mad!

♡ Cotton or any natural fibers. He's organic like that.

♡ No products in the hair and no hooker makeup. Simple is his kind of sexy. In other words, look as close to natural as you can.

♡ A respectable look, like you could be someone's parent. He's got a traditional thing about him.

Tasty Treats

Food

Cancers are finicky about everything, so you can only guess what his eating habits are like. Typically, he's a glutton and lives to eat. However, as much as he loves eating, his tastes buds are completely boring. He's not into trying new things and generally sticks to foods with a sense of familiarity. Forget spicy and exciting; think filling and soothing. Nothing too wacky for him, so make sure places you bring him are cozy and homey, as you don't need him being too overwhelmed and slinking back into his shell before you have a chance to get to know him.

Erotic Eats:

♡ A quiet family-owned home-style-cooking greasy spoon— and can be any ethnicity. He's all about that homey feeling.

♡ Seafood joints. He's a water sign.

♡ Breakfast foods. A twenty-four-hour diner with all-day breakfast is the kind of place he'd find romance in.

♡ Intimate French restaurants. Anything deemed traditionally romantic places for dining will appeal to him.

♡ Places that serve foods you would want to eat if you were home sick—soups, stews, comfort foods, etc. Those foods epitomize his taste.

♡ Lasagna and other things of that consistency and texture— layers of food that are simple and non-complex on the palette. He's typically not a daredevil eater.

♡ Home cooking. He loves the domestic side to love. Show him your stuff in the kitchen or better yet, have him show you his stuff. Cancers usually can cook fairly well.

Movies

Cancer is into being an emotional basket case and can't get enough of loading up on as much drama that'll fit into his bottomless heart. To share a cinematic moment with him, think along the lines of sad, dark, and totally depressing. Pain is beautiful and he loves indulging in it. Anything that brings a viewer through an emotional wringer, with or without the triumphant ending (preferably not), sign him up. Of course, there are those other sides to him and you may as well try to play up to them, too. Comedy and male machismo movies are also his speed, so go for it. He's all for keeping up appearances.

Cinematic Foreplay:

♡ Tearjerkers. Crying and popcorn—totally his type of fun!

♡ Film noir. The darker the better.

♡ Movies with a victorious underdog. Documentary is best, as you can't beat real-life inspiration.

♡ Super-hero action flicks. He'll think he can relate, even if he won't admit to it.

♡ Funny films with lots of physical comedy. He's also one part goofball.

♡ Chick flicks. He's not above it, just as long as you don't tell his friends.

💟 Movies with children in them or family, this could even include mafia/mob movies. He's all for anything family related.

Dating Ideas

In the getting-to-know-you phase, Cancer likes jumping right in. He wants to grab a hold of you, drag you back to his lair, and cuddle up to you—physically, mentally, spiritually, and emotionally. If your energies can flow well in such intimacy, then expect date number two. When he likes you, it means he wants all your attention and needs to give you all of his. He's not one for small talk, so backdrops for your bonding sessions need to offer privacy and, to some extent, a sense of familiarity and calm. If there are others, he'll need the furthest extreme—massive crowds, as he likes blending in and gaining anonymity. When all these pieces of the puzzle fall into place for him to feel at ease, only then can he share who he is: a creative and highly emotional weirdo.

Playful Planning:

💟 A scenic waterfront picnic; don't forget the wine. Anything involving liquids is good with him.

💟 A massage together. Hang at a spa; the soothing environment will bring out his best.

💟 A sporting event. All Cancers have a jock side—even if he denies he's into the whole machismo thing.

💟 Drinking. Cancers enjoy throwing back a few, but beware that they also have a proclivity to being alcoholics. Save yourself the possible heartbreak if you find yourself picking yours up off the floor two hours into your date.

💟 Drumming circles and hippie-dippy things like that. You can never go wrong with a music festival either.

♡ A family get-together. He thrives with that form of social structure.
♡ Any art-related event. This can also mean a craft's fair, as all Cancers have an inner "granny" to them.

Sound Seduction

Conversation

Cancer is a sideways communicator weighted down by massive vulnerabilities. He'll do anything to avoid revealing his own depths early on, preferring to twist conversations to get you to pour your guts out first. He operates better as a listener than a converser, as that's how he endears himself with you. In getting to your nitty-gritty, he assesses his ability to be open with you and your capability to understand and accept his baggage. If you can warm Cancer up, to step out of his shell, he'll gladly pour his guts out and go on and on and on, almost to the extent you wish he'd shut up. Despite his shy come-on, he's an opinionated fucker and will love to jam his thoughts into your head—but only if you're really listening. To Cancer, it's not bonding or interesting unless skeletons come out of the closet.

Icebreakers:

♡ Inquire about his childhood. Cancers are obsessed with their childhood.
♡ Ask family-related questions. It's a subject he can go on and on about—especially his mother. Realize, how he feels and treats her will be the way he'll deal with you.
♡ Ask career-related questions. He's a dreamer and what he does and wants to do may not be the same. Get answers on how big and realistic that disparity is before going any further.
♡ Ask about his pet peeves; he loves to complain.
♡ Ask him about his dream home—what it would look like, where it would be, etc. He's into domestic bliss.

♡ Ask about creative hobbies. He'll have outlets left and right. If he has none, be worried. Cancers need their creative outlets.

♡ Ask where he's lived. Typically, he's been around, as he's obsessed with finding his place.

Music

Music is Cancer's therapy; without it, he'd be consumed by his dark and angry thoughts. It's a prime tool he uses to get his aggressions out and he likes it loud and hard. If he can do some scream therapy with it, even better—'cause God knows, all Cancers need it. Of course, being a sponge for whatever mood is in the air bodes well in using music as a remote control for his emotions. However, he thrives with heavy emotion, angry and soulful. All other moods he'll think are for wimps.

Mood Makers:

♡ Heavy metal, speed metal, hardcore punk, gangsta rap. He digs anything angry and/or aggressive.

♡ Hippie music, psychedelic rock. Music that can put him into a trance works with him.

♡ Eastern spiritual music, chants. He's always down for music that can speak to his higher self.

♡ Classical. It relaxes him and makes him easier to seduce.

♡ Corny retro pop. He's nostalgic and won't be able to deny this.

♡ Classic rock. It helps get him in touch with his masculine side.

♡ Acoustic music. Music from people who sound like they're about to kill themselves or already have is his type of passion.

Gifts

A present symbolizes your love, so it better be meaningful and grand. If not, expect Cancer to be deeply hurt and insulted. Of course, he won't tell you this, but rather he'll internalize the anguish and eventually explode disproportionately at some other random moment. Understand with Cancer, everything you do and say is personal, and a gift is a powerful way to express yourself. Surefire hints that you care include anything handmade, customized, commemorating, expensive, and/or an heirloom. If your present is none of these things, it should at least pamper his soul; anything less will make him feel you think he lacks one—harming him beyond repair.

Boxed Treats:

- ♡ A photo album of your moments together. Sentiment always pulls at his heartstrings.
- ♡ A picture of you as a child. It'll make him endlessly coo.
- ♡ Baked goods or cooking supplies. He loves that Suzie Homemaker crap.
- ♡ Stuff for the bath. He loves taking them.
- ♡ Booze or any mind enhancer. He loves a good escape.
- ♡ Mix CDs made just for him. Personalized gifts rock his soul.
- ♡ Artwork, especially yours. He admires creativity; any expression of yours will be doubly treasured.

Touch Me

The slower you come, the better you'll be. Cancer is a sensualist and everything sexual is better in slow-mo. He likes to feel you out and take his time to absorb the moment. Being that he's in a constant state of self-protection, you have to bare in mind this neurosis and be patient. Even if you've bonded with him quickly, he can still be distant at the snap of a finger. Cancer gets off better when he's eased in and made to feel safe. He's a security hound and a traditionalist at the core, so this means offering up plenty of affection before serving up your meaty smut.

Cancer needs to be warmed up with ambiance and then submerged into a complete scenario. Although he can have his fair share of fast-paced raunch or whatever the mood requires with spontaneous sex, his general preference is for leisurely paced love. This can mean candles, a bubble bath, sultry music, wine, sexy lingerie, flowers. All the elements that can infuse the atmosphere with romance. You can't miss by starting off with a good massage, oils and all. Cancer is naturally adept to give it good and will read your body like braille, drawing all the information and energy he'll need to be the lover you want him to be. Do the same with him and learn every inch of him—as every inch is a g-spot onto itself.

By paying attention to detail, he can gauge the depth of your desires. The level of your reassurance then sets his drive, giving him something to rise to the occasion for or fall short of. Ultimately, what makes him hard and steamy is feeling that his worthiness is appreciated. Plus, being a sentimental guy, he lives seriously, as if every moment is written in stone. By you creating an elaborate stage for your sexual masterpieces, it'll inspire his best performance. So put your all into it and he'll be sure to put his all into you.

Ways to Heat Up Your Cancer:

- ♡ Massage him, concentrate on the upper torso—mostly his chest; it's his pleasure zone. You know it, pinch those nipples!
- ♡ Need him, let him play savior. There's nothing more delicious than sympathy sex from this sweetie. Share your vulnerabilities and let his big hard cock cure all your woes.
- ♡ In public, rub him under the table and play footsie. He likes a good tease before he gets full-on commando on you.
- ♡ Do him near a body of water.
- ♡ Use food erotically, like having him lick flavors off your body. Greet him at the door with his name in chocolate written on you.

♡ Surprise him at home in a flamboyant sexy costume. What he abhors in public, he'll love in private.

♡ Put him in a plush bed—high-thread-count sheets and perhaps a featherbed. The comfort and cuddling alone will be all you need to arouse him.

Role-playing

Cancer has an infinite amount of moods and as many faces, making him one hell of a sexy playmate. Best to create personas that he can inhabit with positivity, as sending him into a dark mode can mean getting him stuck there—and nothing like a sad Cancer to ruin the day. Create uplifting storylines and he'll easily pull the feelings out of him. Then, voila, you're guaranteed for the next few hours (at tops) on the mood he'll be in. As for preferences, let him play out his hero fantasies and show him a "happy ending."

Cast of Characters:

♡ FBI agent taking a defendant away into a witness protection program. All Cancers are into ensuring safety.

♡ Two strangers on a blind date. This gives his imagination free range to go wherever it wants!

♡ Fifth cousins. Yeah, it's sick, but it's the only legal relative this family man has a chance of hooking up with.

♡ Babysitter and parent. Again, it's that tawdry family-man thing, which can include the pervert-dad routine.

♡ Superhero and villain. He'll love saving the day!

♡ World-class athlete and fan. Cancer men all have secret jock fantasies.

♡ Famous historical lovers. Tradition turns him on, so sourcing out an old-fashioned love story will appeal to his idea of gallantry.

Taking the Bait

Cancer goes one way and one way only, and that's right to com-
mitmentville. If you have sex with him, that's pretty much sealing the
deal. Of course, there are those randy Cancers, so make it three
times of hooking up to play it safe. Once the sex part is conquered,
he'll ensue with obvious telltale signs that'll reassure his interest in
being your man. These things will include clearing schedules with
you, sourcing out a routine, and giving you daily calls. He'll fall
right into line with the duties of a boyfriend, as the way Cancer
shows his affection is being possessive and traditional. The more
you respond to him, the more astute he becomes in playing his part.

However, despite his immediate doting lover routine, he'll rarely
be direct in sharing what he wants. He needs to work up to that
because he's got issues. Once he's smitten, eventually his insecurities have to go haywire, as that's the drama he loves and sees as a
part of falling in love. One minute he'll be filled with a feeling of
hopeful exuberance that'll drive him to the heights of romance and
you to cloud nine. Another minute, he'll turn into a defeated old man
who has plummeted to the depths of despair—SOSing to you to pull
him back to safety by professing your affections.

In playing these games, Cancer's working out his place in your
heart and finding your place in his. You can call him on it, but no
matter what you say, he still has to go through his process. Then,
even after going through those tests, there's still that one last trial to
seal the deal: Meeting his family and mother will be your judgment
day. Whether he loves or loathes her, he's haunted by her. Save
yourself the aggravation and bond with her the best you can or suffer the consequences.

Not being a halfway guy, Cancer has to prove your connection
is a worthwhile investment through and through. If you've jumped all
the hurdles correctly, you'll know for sure when he sets future plans
into motion. As soon as he trusts his feelings and yours, he'll fall into

place and do all the things a future family man would do. So, while there may be massive amounts of turmoil to get you to this moment, know the flip side is that he's looking to love, honor, and cherish you until death do you part.

UNAUTHORIZED: ASTRAL AUTOPSY

Recognizing Fear

Cancer is obsessed with security. It either makes him a complete loner or a co-dependent freak. It's most evident with the way he spends money. To prepare for disaster, he lives with the threat of catastrophe hanging over his shoulder and is always saving for that rainy day. It's the paranoia that inspires Cancer's cautiously anal behavior and can possibly turn him into a hermit. At least if he does the latter, he saves others from dealing with his insanities.

Main cause
Always seeing the glass half-empty.

Immunizing His Fears:

- ♡ Nurture the hell out of him and never judge his feelings.
- ♡ Always double-, triple-check the doors are locked. Seeing you also have this compulsion will put him at ease about his security concerns.
- ♡ Know karate or learn some kind of self-defense. It'll ease his mind to know you can protect him.
- ♡ When he calls, try to pick up on the first or second ring every time or he'll think you don't love him.
- ♡ Don't share him, to the point of obsession. Be extremely possessive. For example, if you're in an elevator, press CLOSE DOOR

quickly. If someone tries to get in and gets the door shut in their face, you'll both have a good laugh together that'll bring you closer with love. He's all about the one-on-one time in every sense of the word.

Infecting Him with Fear:

- ♡ Be loud in public and cause attention to be cast upon the two of you.
- ♡ Wake him up in the middle of the night to ask if he's locked the door.
- ♡ Drain his phone battery and yours before hitting the road and then go, "Oops," when you're forty-five minutes into your trip. Also, pack no food or water for the ride.
- ♡ Be belligerent to authority figures. He has issues with them.
- ♡ Tailgate as if your bumper were made of magnets.

Recognizing Anger

If there's any emotion this guy is in touch with, it's his anger. Everything pisses Cancer off and he has no problem expressing it, except to the source of his contention. Convinced he's got all the answers to life, if anyone deters from his law, he'll then despise that person with every cell in his body, for all of eternity—as that's the pain he feels when people "disrespect" his unspoken rules. Plus, it's not only that he'll get mad and say nothing, he'll hold on to that grudge and then act out without anyone understanding why. Sure you can give in, but then he won't respect you. The fact is there's no winning with Cancer.

Main cause
Being passive-aggressive and conflicted with a fascist's point of view.

Immunizing His Anger:

- ♡ Leave him alone. Anger is his guilty pleasure and he's going to indulge in it no matter what, because being mad makes him feel tough.
- ♡ Mock him sweetly. Self-deprecating humor is his schtick.
- ♡ Always remember to say thank you.
- ♡ Be angrier than him—like with road rage, scream insanely at drivers from your window, even if you're just a passenger. Over-the-top behavior balances him out.
- ♡ Get him fucked up or feed him. Make it easy on yourself by pacifying him.

Infecting Him with Anger:

- ♡ In front of his friends, pull up in a car and pull away when he goes for the door. Even the most innocent humiliations will scour his soul.
- ♡ Insult his family in any way. Go for the Mom if you want to go for the jugular. It won't matter if he loves or loathes her, either; no one can say anything, but him, about Mother.
- ♡ Talk to him during a movie, but ignore him while he tries to talk to you.
- ♡ Engage strangers in conversations, everywhere you go. He's typically too antisocial to deal.
- ♡ Go out and come back with something to drink or eat for you, but nothing for him—and don't acknowledge you've ignored asking him if he wanted anything.

Recognizing Sadness

Cancer is the moodiest sign of the zodiac and holds a Ph.D. in depression. He's the guy who likes diving into all the shades of gray. As a scholar of the grim, no one, at least in his mind, can compare to the sadness he feels because he's so "sensitive." However, what he might define as sensitive, others might define as sourpuss behavior. Sure, there are times he'll see a silver lining—but generally, his attitude is: Why bother setting yourself up for a letdown?

Main cause
He believes that pain makes him grow.

Immunizing His Sadness:

♡ Feed him a grand-fest of dull foods. Domestic bliss is his paradise.

♡ Indulge him, cry with him. If you both do it, it's romantic, not sad.

♡ Never bring up an ex with any happy memory attached. Everyone compared to him must be considered a total loser.

♡ Put up lots of framed pictures of happy moments in his life. He thrives with nostalgia.

♡ Create traditions with him. Personal celebrations are what make relationships special.

Infecting Him with Sorrow:

♡ When you bump into someone you know, don't introduce him. Sure, this bothers everyone, but it burns Cancer.

♡ Whenever he cooks, say you already ate. You can also pick at it, too. Reject his cooking; reject him.

♡ Behave poorly around children. He'll feel protective, even if he doesn't really like them.

♡ Leave him alone for a few hours; he'll be sure to find a bad mood to sink into all by himself.

♡ Ask to see his baby picture and then laugh hysterically at it. His inner child is already wounded enough; your laughter will be more daggers to his heart.

Recognizing Trust

It takes forever for Cancer to trust, unless you're his mother. For the normal person who didn't squeeze him out of her vagina, winning his trust can be an uphill struggle. Even so, there are only degrees of trust he'll readily offer up and all of it can be withdrawn at a moment's notice. So, unless you're able to hypnotize him into thinking you'll never ever hurt him or even mildly offend him, realize he'll always have a suspicious nature. His belief: You can never be too careful.

Main cause
You can't be a real mama's boy, unless she's the only one you trust.

Immunizing Him with Trust:

♡ Make his birthday a big deal, despite his endless protests against making it into an event.

♡ Be able to see past his moodiness and accept that's him. Unconditional love or bust!

♡ Remember things like his grandfather's favorite pie. This will impress him blind. Showing interest in his family will automatically score you major points.

♡ Put money periodically into your savings account. How you budget is a sign of character.

♡ Keep every morsel of memorabilia. Being excessively sentimental makes him trust you more. His logic: If you're a sap like him, you're okay.

Infecting His Sense of Trust:

♡ Give him the same lame present twice. He won't trust anything you do is personal after that.

♡ Answer your phone when you're with him, but talk in another room. He'll think you're talking about him.

- ♡ Lie to your mother and have him overhear. If you can lie to her, you can lie to anyone.
- ♡ Forget to lock his door once. He'll forever see you as absent-minded.
- ♡ Always be happy. He won't understand you; therefore, he will be unable to trust you.

Recognizing Motivation

Cancer is a dreamer. His aspirations border on the fantastical, and when mixed with his delicate temperament, any hint of failure can cause him to retreat. This is why it's essential to coddle him into playing the hero. Yes, motivate him by giving him a chance to be a martyr and going into action for someone else or a team, better yet his family. Not that he's isn't self-obsessed, because he is, but when it comes to protecting and comforting others, he'll be much quicker to the draw.

Main cause
What would he have to complain about, if there were no expectations placed on him?

Immunizing His Motivation

- ♡ Tell him you had a bad premonition about whatever circumstance is in question. He's a believer in signs.
- ♡ Comfort is the best Cancer de-motivator. If you want him to stay put, do it with food, a TV, and a couch.
- ♡ Deflate his spirit by being rigid, uncreative, logical, or competitive. He's at his best in an imaginative and casual setting.
- ♡ Throw a spotlight on him whenever you want him to cool it, unless he's already in his super spazzy mode. If that's the case, steal his audience.
- ♡ Act like his mother. His instinctive reaction will be to rebel and do the opposite.

Infecting Him with Motivation:

- ♡ Mother his needs and aspirations, but don't baby him.
- ♡ Send in a kid to ask him your favor. He has a soft spot for children.
- ♡ He'd do anything to ensure safety for himself and his loved one. If you need him to do something, say it'll make you feel "safer."
- ♡ Create a family dynamic with him. He thrives on this environment.
- ♡ If you can save him money, he'll do anything to keep that extra dime in his pocket.

DESTINATION: DUMPSVILLE

Celestial Voodoo on You

Like his shellfish cousin the clam, Cancer slams shut as soon as he's been touched in a way he doesn't approve—and once he closes, it's final. He's an unforgiving fucker and once you hurt him, forget it. Even worse, a majority of the times you can offend him without even being aware of it. Sure, you can try to squeeze out his feelings, but if you're already dealing with him on the defensive, then you're playing to lose. He'll lay the guilt on so thick; he'll look to break you. It's not just that you apologize profusely, it's that you show him your pain—as that's what he gets off on. The more you have made him suffer, multiply that times twenty and that's what he wants you to feel. Plead all you want, but all he'll do is savor your anguish and hold his grudge tighter.

If you happen to not be what he's looking for and have been nothing but pleasant, then your demise will be a bit different. It'll be based on his guilt and he'll start treating you like a terminally ill patient as soon as it's apparent to him that he can't go on. Just when you start thinking his kindness is a sign that your bond is intensifying, he'll start to crack and blindside you with a breakup. Yeah, either way he goes, it all winds up bad, because he's clumsy dealing with his emotions and being that he just can't communicate, it means hellish breakups that'll drag in more drama than necessary. So, if he isn't declaring his undying love to you every day and being somewhat of a doormat, then realize your days may be numbered. Even not, it's anyone's guess. He's unpredictable and too moody for words. Sure, he likes to settle in and down, but he also loves drama. So, unless you're a mind reader and can control the universe, forget trying to pinpoint where he's going and appreciate the times you've already shared.

. . . And Other Signs He Hates You

He shares a name with a deadly and contentious disease—that alone says something. However, the survival rate for the illness is probably higher than the Crab's forgiveness rate. To say the least, when Cancer hates you, it's forever. Basically walking around with a tension that can snap at any time, look at Cancer wrong on his off days and he might punch you out. Hate is never far from the surface and anything that rubs him the wrong way leaves a deep impression. He's an angry fucker and his disdain is doled out quite generously.

When enraged, he'll turn into the most judgmental bastard you've ever met. In public, he won't acknowledge you, and to anyone that knows you, he'll drop the 4-1-1 on your immorality as if you were a carcinogen. Ninety-nine percent of the times it's way more consuming for him than it is for you, being that he refrains from communicating to you. While everyone else might know why you're on his shit list, you might never find out. It makes it easy for you to cast him off as nuts, as he bastes in his angst like a dirty diaper. Sure, you can fall into the guilt and care, but why bother? There are too many fishes in the sea to have to torture yourself over this immature a-hole.

Beating Him to the Punch

It typically takes only one good shot to his ego to get Cancer to slink away. He's so sensitive that even a slight threat of humiliation can make him melt—but, of course, there are those stubborn ones that have a high threshold of pain and get off on guilting people. This Cancer will do anything to win back your love or die trying. If you happen to be stuck with one, there's only one way to get rid of him, and that's sadistically.

Start off by getting bossy and withholding the sex. Stick to the chores and get him to clean your fridge, re-tar your driveway, and scrub your toilets. Only after your house is cleaned, his hands cal-lused, and you haven't fucked him in forever will he start to get the hint that he's been used—but only maybe. He does believe in pain as a way to gain, so with this breakup, you never know how low he'll keep sinking. The deeper his worship, the more relentless he'll be to hold on. Only when he hits rock bottom and sees you as a total fucker will he be able to reconcile his feelings. Otherwise, he'll always dig for an ounce of hope. With him, it's love or hate, no in between. So, to say the least, it can get ugly when you hit the finale.

Overall, Cancer's attitude underneath it all is that life's a letdown. After he's gets a good look at his depravity, he'll save face by put-ting on his brave look and go back in his hole to suffer in silence. However, he'll be angrier and hold his emotions in even tighter. You almost do him a favor by validating his negativity and should walk away patting yourself on the back. His life's mission is to prove it sucks, and your assault on his emotions only verifies his self-fulfilling prophecy.

Ridding Yourself of Cancer with Minimal Scarring:

- ♡ Humiliate him. Make fun of his manhood in public.
- ♡ Get him into a mindless fight and leave it at that. He might never return, as his pride bruises easily.
- ♡ Insult his family. Be warned, he might hate you for life for this one. He's a staunch family man.
- ♡ Be overly social without him or leave him to have to be social without you. It's like leaving a non-swimmer out in the ocean.
- ♡ Be friends with your ex and hang with him frequently. The jealousy will consume Cancer.
- ♡ Be super moody, more so than him. He can dish it out, but he can't take it.
- ♡ Be too nice to him. More chances than not, Cancer feels so "damaged" that he won't know what to do when treated like a human being.

Kick, Drop, and Kill

A bad experience with Cancer ages you, even if you only dated for a week. It's stressful because this fucker knows how to go deep inside and turn screws. He'll play you like a piano, bringing out your most profoundly beautiful music to the most terrifyingly dark melodies that'll haunt you infinitely. After all, this is how he operates, so it's only natural to suck you in the turmoil that is his reality. Being around Cancer inevitably turns your perspective on yourself inside out—showing you the depraved levels you'd go for love and also the selfless sacrifices you'd make. It brings out your best and worst emotions, as he's a mirror for souls who wish to look in.

If you can take this experience for what it's worth and rise past the giant mind-fuck that leaves you with more questions than answers, you can come out the winner. In the end, best to rely on your own intuition to gauge who won the battles, but if you've come out alive and are able to walk away, then you most certainly have won the war. The irony is that the reality of it all was staring you in the face all the while. True to his symbol the crab, it may have taken a lot of work and a little bloodshed to yank out that minuscule piece of meat inside this slippery sucker, but damn it, the taste is so impossibly delicious that the pain almost seems worth it.

WANTED: LEO

Chivalrous spendthrift with a megawatt smile known to blind onlookers to his egotistically controlling clutches. Turn on a spotlight and he will appear.

BARE BASICS

How to Spot Him

There are men in this world who have the power to make individuals swoon with just a flash of their smile. These men are recognizable as soon as they enter a room. He'll have a sublime gait that'll melt you with his motions, tantalizing you into a sexy daydream and making you deliriously docile. The more you admire him, the more indescribable the sensations and you'll greedily need to know more. Even if you don't get close enough, just the gaze as he saunters by will leave an impression deep in you, as just that one second can bring you into a silent submission as if God were in the air.

Welcome to Leo, the swashbuckler, the sex symbol, and the superstar. He's born with a captivating quality that not even science can explain, and his magnetism draws in the masses to worship at his feet without much effort on his part. He has a confident aura about him that makes the world spin around him at an exciting pace with onlookers seeking out his approval. The good thing, though, is that he's usually a benevolent ruler and is always seeking to create good times for as many as possible. Plus, he has no trouble taking responsibility for that fun, either, as he's a generous individual with deep pockets and will stop at nothing to keep the festive spirit alive. Yes, with Leo in the room, there's always a celebration to be had and done up as extravagantly as possible.

The thing with Leo, though, is he comes in several varieties. Symbolized by the lion, Leo will take on a felinesque manner that can manifest in various ways. There's the King Sheba Leo, who needs to be in control, the bob cat Leo, who needs to play, and then there's the pussycat Leo, who can be fussy and needs independence. However, all three will have a big ego that needs to be stroked on a regular basis, as he's fueled by idol worship. As a natural-born performer, Leo will soak in the spotlight anyway it comes. To ensure it, he'll play up to whatever environment he's in and charismatically wrestle who he desires under his control. It's not that he just wants to be liked; he needs to be lavished with love—and by everyone.

If you happen to cross his path while he's on the prowl for some tail, expect Leo to be more so in his prime. He'll have all his feathers out, ruling the scene and making his grand-prize status obvious. However, despite the big show, the deal is that Leo is a big ole traditional romantic at heart, looking to find a love so big, so pure, so passionate, and so inspiring that it'll redefine the concept of love for the world, throughout all time. If you think this sounds like a tall order, then move on. For Leo, only idealistic lovers who strive for the fantastical need apply.

Key Features:

- ♡ Hair! Usually he's sporting a thick mane with a superb style. If he's lost some, he'll still have a head worth fondling
- ♡ A sunny disposition marked by a big wide toothy grin
- ♡ Regal stance and good posture
- ♡ Smooth steady strut, a felinesque way about his moves

♡ A loud presence, either via voice and/or appearance—like loud clothes, out-of-control hair, and/or strong aura; possibly even an overly potent perfumed scent

♡ Found in the center of a group, rarely alone

♡ The generous guy with the deep wallet

Seducing Him into Your Boudoir

If you want him, then you better have balls. Leo doesn't humble himself for second best, so rule #1: Be comfortable in your own skin. He thinks himself as royalty and seeks an equal. If he senses any shame, you may as well demote yourself to peasant slut because that's where he'll put you. With Leo, how you feel about yourself, present yourself, and price yourself as a trophy piece all matter—so leave the modesty act behind.

The fact is you don't have to be the prettiest, smartest, sexiest, or the most successful to bag a Leo, although those qualities help to back you up. With Leo, it's all in your attitude to think yourself the best. Act as if the sun rises and sets with you and you've won half the battle for his attention. The other half is making him feel like he's the light of the universe and possibly the most important being ever. Yes, flattery matters, but draw the line just short of gushing. Although Leo does love the fanfare, he won't stand for groveling. Respect is the key word. Have it for yourself and for him. Know how to be smooth and hold court over your emotions early on.

If Leo wants you, all you should have to do is flash an enticing sexy glance and cheeky smile. This will send him into a primal mode to track your scent and give him his bearings as the dominant one (his preferred role) as he sniffs his way to you. Then, in his presence, enthrall him with confident conversation or show off seductive dance moves. The more alluring your impression, the higher he'll go to prove himself worthy—which is exactly where you want him. Leo loves a good chase and a chance to display the highest levels of his charisma. Ensure this by making every aspect of the courtship worthy of a romance novel, even down to the part when you let him take you in his arms to whisk you away into the sunset.

Loving Him in the Boudoir

He's a demon in the sack. Leo's got charisma, passion, enthusiasm, stamina, imagination, and lots of spontaneity—plus, he'll shower you with all the attention to make you feel as if he's absolutely and insanely in love with you.

Leo isn't the guy who undresses you, uses you, and falls asleep. He's way too dramatic and romantic for that! Think of each encounter like a soap opera episode, sultry scenes taking on many dimensions, but an energy that's always of romance. It's his aim to make love. At his most ungraceful, he'll just give sex. If he's looking to impress, however, he'll go into his over-the-top hot-throbbing porn-star fuck mode. Sex is Leo's ultimate feel-good activity, and he wants his lovers to feel good about themselves and him—and of course, he wants to feel good, too. This only works when everyone is feeling their most stunning, and he guarantees it. If he has to blow smoke up your ass to get you to that state, he'll pour on the compliments until you're giddy. Use this knowledge to your advantage, as getting lost in it is great; but if you're playing to win, always up the ante. If you don't make him earn you, know that when he's pumping you, he's really pumping himself. So, work it to bring out the best in him.

The most delicious thing about Leo sex is once you get him where you want he's powerfully present every time he pulls out the love rod, always striving for the gold. Everything will matter, as he takes in all the ambiance to direct his scenes. Then, once the action starts rolling, expect him to take the lead (which makes it fabulous for anyone that likes being a bottom). Leo is all about proving his virility, and that'll mean taking you into the palm of his hands to make you

ooze under the force of his manhood. Throw in a few verbal compliments after the heat of passion, like how you never saw such a
big cock or that you never came like that before, and he'll gladly do
it all over again.

MAKING HIM COME TO THE
PALM OF YOUR HAND

Eye Candy

The man is gaudy. Leo lives to lavish himself with attention in any
way he can. Being loudly dressed is a neon sign that he's in the
room, and a marker for where the spotlight should be directed.
Give him a rise by following suit: outrageous costumes that show off
your uniqueness or classic styles that reek of fashion and expense.
Top it with your crowning glory as your jewel because he just loves
hair. Then, count your minutes until he swoops you under his gaze
and ravishes you bottom to top. Just one vital fact to address, however: Whatever your show-stopping style, remember he's the star
and you're the supporting cast.

Stylin' Seduction:

♡ Vibrant colors: red, gold, orange, and yellow. They're all
   Leo's signature colors.
♡ Hats or anything that draws attention to your hair. Makeup is
   also welcome; anything theatrical in any sense of the word is
   a turn-on for this one.
♡ Have good hair, styled up the wazoo or just really healthy
   and shiny.
♡ Good shoes with a nice heel. This helps keep your posture
   statuesque.

♡ Expensive labels. Status matters.
♡ Flamboyance. Take risks and go as far off the edge as you want. He loves anyone that can pull off courageous fashions.
♡ Animal prints. The louder, the better—but style them right or risk looking ridiculous.

Tasty Treats

Food

Leos don't skimp, especially when it comes to food. He's got a big appetite and is addicted to overindulgence. Load him up with the crème de la crème, as he'll swallow nothing less—and keep the portions large because his eyes are bigger than his stomach. Toss in a dash of spicy drama and sweet romance to the experience, and you'll have a perfectly simmered Leo sauntering into your clutches. Be decadent, in every sense of the word, as that's the way Leo licks it.

Erotic Eats:

♡ Smoked or BBQ foods. Anything that requires flames, serve it up! He's a fire sign and Leos all love fired-up foods.
♡ Spicy foods. The hotter the better.
♡ Expensive food. Champagne, lobster, filet mignon, caviar, etc. He's the original surf-and-turf date.
♡ Dinner theater. Mix together drama and food, and that spells yum to a Leo.
♡ To be seen places. This can include trendy hot spots, places where you might see a celeb or even a celebrity chef restaurant to sample the tasting menu.
♡ A catered dinner in a stretch limo as it drives around town. Use your imagination with him for dining experiences that are flamboyant and original.
♡ A dinner party. He loves any place he'll have an audience.

Movies

The first thing to consider when going to the movies with Leo is the screen, because size matters. The larger it is the bigger his excitement, because being overwhelmed captures his attention and imagination—so, go as wide and long as possible. As for content, he has a penchant for explosive action, high drama, passionate romance, and burning emotions. Anything over the top will be grand. One warning, though: Leo is the sign that rules entertainment; choose wisely as selecting a dud will reflect poorly upon you.

Cinematic Foreplay:

- ♡ Big action with major special effects. He likes to be transported into the plot.
- ♡ The blockbusters of the moment: domestic or international. He always wants to know what the top things are.
- ♡ Biographical movies on famous people. He'll take notes and compare himself to them.
- ♡ Musicals with dance numbers. It's over-the-top entertainment at its finest!
- ♡ Movies with kids in them. Leo is the sign that rules children and has a soft spot for them, even if he doesn't want any of his own.
- ♡ Romantic comedies. He's the sign of romance.
- ♡ Super hi-fi drama with total tearjerker power. Yes, he's the sign that rules drama.

Dating Ideas

He'll do anything, as long as someone's watching. After all, Leo is on 24-7. Take him to the center of it all, where there's action, excitement, and/or a party atmosphere, and he'll be in his element. He's an adventurer and loves to charge his adrenaline. Plus, with you as his cheerleader, he'll feel extra self-assured and thrive on showing off his charms. So, put him on a stage, and he'll gladly entertain you for hours, as the only way to really learn who he is and what he's all about is by admiring him.

Playful Planning:

- ♡ Karaoke. He loves the spotlight and hamming it up, even if bestowed with the most dreadful voice.
- ♡ Tickets to see a live taping of a TV show. Anything involving entertainment and its industry is his thing.
- ♡ Rock climbing or anything involving a mountain or a bit of danger. The great outdoors makes him thrive.
- ♡ Out in the sun anywhere, doing anything. The sun is his ruler.
- ♡ A casino. He loves to take big risks.
- ♡ Dancing, going to a nightclub or a place with live music. Action and lights turn him on.
- ♡ A party. He loves meeting new people, and being in a crowd gives him something to do: look to stand out and take over.

Sound Seduction

Conversation

No matter what he's saying, Leo delivers his words with a sense of importance. In his mind, there's always a spotlight on him with inquiring minds needing to know. His pride is always on the line, so be prepared to feel like a casting director as he gives his mono-logue. With this known, realize Leo likes intense topics—giving him the best fuel for soliloquies. Lead him to the grandiose or controversial and watch him go. Just be warned, he loves compelling dialogue and if that means exaggerating a tale or two, oh well. Not to say he's prone to lying, but he loves to keep his audience entertained.

Icebreakers:

♡ Ask him about his past love affairs. Know who you're dealing with right off the bat. Besides, he loves talking about love.

♡ Discuss the best performances he has been to. What was his first? These will be his top memories.

♡ Ask what his first kiss was like. Get his romantic quotient.

♡ If he could be any celebrity, who would he be and why? You can gauge his depth from this answer.

♡ Talk about art. Ask what his favorite pieces are, in any medium. Leos are artistically inclined.

♡ Find out his biggest accomplishment to date. See how big his ego really is.

♡ Find out about his most risqué sex/love moment. See what you're in for.

Music

Leo is always in the mood for a party, and nothing sets the mood better than the right music. So, create your moments with songs that properly set your festivities in motion. Just choose your atmosphere: intimate, raunchy, festive, etc. If you hit the right notes, then he'll keep you dazzled all night long. Turn him on by turning up the ecstasy music, and infuse the ambiance with sounds that make him feel like God. Music themes that resonate extravagance, romance, passion, pain, fury, madness, beauty, and/or desperation will be superb. Plus, if it's got a good beat, slip it on in.

Mood Makers:

♡ Large orchestral music. He loves anything grandiose.

♡ Opera. It's uber-dramatic, which is his mode.

♡ Classic hard rock. Long guitar solos bring out his inner rock star.

♡ Love songs. He's the sign that rules romance.

♡ Funk. If it's gritty and sexy, even better!

♡ Sleek overproduced music that sounds expensive. Anything polished and costly is good with him.

♡ Glam rock or any band with a flamboyant look and sound. Again, over-the-top things are his taste.

Gifts

The bigger the box, the sweeter the prize. Who even cares what's in the package, as anything big impresses Leo. If it happens to be in a tiny package, then you better make sure it comes with a big price tag. When shopping for this Grandmaster of Flash, realize his tastes are more extravagant than the norm. If you spot something you think is offensively tacky that you can't take your eyes off of, rest assured you probably just hit a gold mine of a gift for Leo. Ostentation isn't just welcome; it's a prerequisite for his perfect present.

Boxed Treats:

♡ Something for his entertainment system, like, say, his own karaoke machine. Get ready with the earplugs, though.

♡ A surprise party. Nothing beats a roomful of worshippers.

♡ Front-row concert tickets. He'd rather be on the stage, but this will do.

♡ A day at a spa. He's good at getting pampered.

♡ Art. Either something you've made with him as your muse or something you thought represented him. Feed his ego sweetly.

♡ Jewelry with a monogram professing your worship. He loves having his territory defined.

♡ BBQ equipment. No, not the most romantic present, but something any Leo will love.

Touch Me

Leo likes it on top. Some may think this is control-freak behavior, but he's filled with so much sexual energy and enthusiasm that he can't contain himself and can't help but want to pounce when he gets hot. After all, he's the lion and will have a jungle-cat quality about him. As his lucky pleasure prey, the only things you need to do when it comes down to it is to look pretty and have fun.

However, to bring out the best sex in him, there are a few tricks. The first thing to note is that he takes a primal approach to his conquests. This means having discipline to tame his bestial side and make him drool with desire before feeding yourself to him. Otherwise, he'll gorge himself sick and not want the taste anymore. Be smart: Teach him portion control by sharing, not handing yourself over to him. He takes his role as a man seriously and where he marks his territory must be a place worthy of his crown jewels. So do your part and show off your self-respect, but don't be shy about also revealing your sex-starved maniac side that can go head to head with what he's got. That's right, get him curious, make him burn with a passionate intensity and want to stop at nothing to get satisfaction, as earning his keep is the way of his pride.

With Leo, everything is foreplay; throw in the drama and put out the hoops for him to jump through. They'll be as effective as a noose around his neck, enhancing his pleasure before emission. Having a performer's mentality, he needs an entire scenario, not just the act of sex, to get him off. Then, when it's actual booty time, don't hold back! Let loose your abandon and go wild. He likes lovers with spirit and ones who are confident to show their passion for him and for sex in general. He thrives on sex that's physically overwhelming. Stroke him everywhere. Every inch of his body is fair game. Express your lust by matching his creativity and enthusiasm and watch him purr with desire. Also note, he's a man driven by his ego, so satisfying you will be necessary for his own gratification. To ensure you always get his prime meat, periodically up the ante on the sexual intensity. Challenge inspires him and he'll push harder to show he's boss and prove to you that being on your knees is a delicious place to be.

Ways to Heat Up Your Leo:

♡ Just like a kitty, Leo loves to get his back massaged, scratched, and rubbed. Give him a back massage, then his head, then his ego, and then his other head.

♡ Do him somewhere you might get an audience, like a balcony or a glass elevator.

♡ Lick him suggestively.

♡ Break out the lights and camera. He'll be ready for his close-up.

♡ Play his machismo card. Let others try to win you over, but let him know who you truly desire. Nothing is hotter for him than to think he's won some cockfight.

♡ Do him with style: in a pricey hotel in a plush bed (the higher the sheet's thread count, the better he'll perform). Or nab him in a limo with champagne and caviar waiting. All Leos have rock star fantasies.

♡ Do him in nature. Try somewhere majestic, like a mountaintop.

Role-playing

Hamming it up gets Leo hot. Add in an erotic flavor to the scene and this man will take it to the next level. Typecast him with parts where he gets to be the hero, the star, the protagonist; make him into the one nobody can keep their eyes off and the one everybody wants to put their hands on. There's no limit to how outrageous the storyline can be, either; as long as you've got extreme emotions and antics he'll give you a performance worthy of an Oscar.

Cast of Characters:

- ♡ Rock star and groupie. It's his version of feeling godlike.
- ♡ Movie producer and budding star on the casting couch. Leo rules the entertainment industry.
- ♡ Characters from his favorite movies. He'll love playing the leading man.
- ♡ A royal couple. This will allow him to indulge his delusions of grandeur.
- ♡ Texas oil baron and stripper. Who is more over the top than a Texan oil baron?
- ♡ Lion tamer and lion. Hello, he is the lion sign.
- ♡ Jet-set playboy and centerfold. This is a variation of the decadent lifestyle idea he loves.

Taking the Bait

Being single isn't Leo's style. After all, how can he gauge his fabulousness without someone worshipping him? Or distinguish himself as a leader, unless there's at least one person seeking his approval? Sure, it's a tad egotistical, but this is Leo. If you can accept and embrace that fact, then you've got the bait he's hungry for. Not to say this is a thankless job, as the perks are top shelf. Lucky are you if you're the object of Leo's affections.

As the ruler of romance, he spares no expense to seal the deal, and there's no denying Leo's emotions. He's over the top by nature, knowing no limits in showering you with love, gifts, and insanely delicious adulation. He'll do anything to spoil you silly. He'll have you believing the love you share spins the world round, as romance is his inspiration and helps bring out his selfless and invincible side. As his muse, he'll be unrelenting in showing you his gratitude. If you want to mark the level at which he loves you, just check the receipts. He's the guy who puts his money where his heart is.

Yes, being loved by Leo can be likened to winning a game show—complete with the grand announcement, a flood of fanfare, and extreme prizes. When in love, he's consumed by it and wants to share it with everyone. He'll brag about you, show you off all over town, and want to spend every minute with you or dreaming of you. Expect only his best behavior, too: an absolute gentleman ensuring you the red-carpet treatment everywhere you go. In fact, he'll be a tyrant about others respecting you, defending your honor in any way possible.

As the original Mr. Chivalry/Captain of the Universe, the place Leo will be most ardent about his affections for you will be with his circle. As a believer in hierarchies, he'll rank you second in his chain of command. With his unspoken code of deference, his cronies will then be required to also bow down to you. If there's disobedience, the penalty is discharge. He likes to keep a tight ship, and if someone falls out of line, he has no problem making him or her walk the plank. Once you've hit this extreme brand of devotion with Leo, you have indeed hit his jackpot of love.

UNAUTHORIZED: ASTRAL AUTOPSY

Recognizing Fear

Pride is Leo's kryptonite. Keeping up appearances is everything to him and he'll do anything to preserve it. If things start to crack and undermine his greatness, the sweat will pour. (Psychologically, that is; forget waiting for him to look anything less than cool.) He hates uncertainty and the threat of embarrassment. While he loves the spotlight, he doesn't like it when it's turned around on him and possibly showing him as a fool. Of course, being such cocky individual, egg on his face will be an inevitable fact of life.

Main cause
Humiliation.

Immunizing His Fears:

♡ Throw him a party or take him to one. What can ever go wrong at a party?

♡ Be co-dependent. He loves having someone there 24-7.

♡ Be his opposite and have a different career and/or hobbies. He hates to feel as if he has to compete with you. It's a stress he could live without.

♡ Drag in extra drama to oversaturate an already tense situation to bring him back around. If you freak out more, he'll have to balance you out and be the hero.

♡ Be a good listener. He hates to fight for his turn to talk.

Infecting Him with Fear:

♡ Pretend not to notice when he becomes anxious—which will be obvious. He won't be smiling much and will show a slight deer-in-the-headlights stare periodically. He'll feel alone and too proud to ask for your nurturance. Dealing with anything alone freaks him out.

♡ Subtly let him know you had an ex who was super gorgeous, successful, and charming. The threat of this man reappearing will intimidate the hell out of him.

♡ If he's picked out a stunning outfit for some big fete he's looking forward to, tell him you heard someone else is going to wear the same thing.

♡ Secretly call up a men's hair club and put his name on the mailing list. Upon receiving the mail, he'll be freaked. Even if he's not losing it, he'll consider it an omen. Sure, all men worry about hair loss, but none like Leo—the sign of hair.

♡ Give compliments to others you know he'll think are lame and then compliment him in the same manner. This will make him fearful that your judgment is completely off.

Recognizing Anger

Forget to bow down and feel his wrath. Disrespect is the biggest faux pas in Leo's world and brings him over the edge. He's a stickler for being treated as if he were God, and his patience is delicate. If you do offend him, most minor charges will be given one calm warning of disdain, but that's it. If you then choose to again deter from his golden rule of reverence, expect to hear his roar. However, despite his anger coming on quick and suddenly, keep in mind that his bark is usually bigger than his bite.

Main cause
Disrespect.

Immunizing His Anger:

♡ Always give direct eye contact when he talks, giving that due respect keeps him in check.

♡ Give him a back massage and turn him into your putty.

♡ Don't be short on the compliments, but don't go overboard. He wants to trust your opinion, not get his ass blatantly kissed.

♡ When playing games with him, be a gracious winner.

♡ Allow him the spotlight, unless he openly concedes it to you.

Infecting Him with Anger:

♡ Put up unattractive pictures of him on your wall when you're planning to have guests over.

- ♡ Put him on hold for too long or take other calls over him during times outside of work.
- ♡ Compliment his enemy. True loyalty means hating who he hates.
- ♡ If there's food on his face, toilet paper stuck on his shoe or hanging out of his pants, don't tell him, but rather tell another person you're with and snicker. Any form of public humiliation will cause his wrath to unfold.
- ♡ Mess with his hair or any of his hair products.

Recognizing Sadness

Leo feels intensely; his sadness equals manic depression. Yes, even the smallest things can create these major dramas, making it hard to gauge when to take it seriously. Generally, if he's really in a self-doubting rut, he'll go into solitude, as he hates for anyone to see him in less than superstar mode. If he's out and about with the pity party, realize it's just a ploy for extra praise. Throw some love his way and cure his blues. Yes, even the life of the party has to crash every now and then.

Main cause
Sorrow is just another brand of drama and he likes showing off his versatility.

Immunizing His Sadness:

- ♡ Get him dolled up and dress up for him. Nothing makes someone happier than being pretty or being around someone who is.
- ♡ Always have presents for him, little tokens of your affection: cupcakes, a mix CD, a framed photo of the two of you, etc. Leo thrives being loved like an idol.

♡ Touch him often. Physicality is essential to his care.

♡ Get your friends to adore him, too. Acceptance from everyone you know is as important as your love.

♡ When in the car, sing along with him, but always let him have the lead.

Infecting Him with Sorrow:

♡ Tell him he reminds you of a famous celeb and then reveal a lame B-list one.

♡ Only want to hang out with him one-on-one in private places. Leo needs fanfare or else.

♡ When he gets a haircut or has on a new outfit, don't acknowledge it.

♡ Choose your friends over him. He's #1 or bust.

♡ Don't seek his approval. Although Leo admires people who are incredibly independent, he doesn't want to sleep next to them.

Recognizing Trust

Loyalty is his trust and the pillar for his most important relationships. Leo will be select with who he gives it to because it takes time and/or DNA for him to grant it (his suspicious mind thinks everybody wants something from him). Even if he has nothing, he'll still find something he'll imagine you want from him. It's not like he doesn't want to share, but you're never in the clear until you perform some grand gesture of humbling admiration he can respect you for. Yes, trust means believing in his insane image he has of himself and defending it as if it were your own.

Main cause

If you support his ego long enough, you're in.

Immunizing His Trust:

♡ Be generous back. Prove you're no freeloader.

♡ Take pride in yourself. Having vanity shows you know how to play the game and proves you'll be an asset to him.

♡ Be passionate and creative. Without that, he'll think you're dull and he'd be damned to trust someone boring!

♡ Exude success. Survival of the fittest is his motto.

♡ Bow to all his demands. A person without a backbone can't be trusted in times of need. If you can't be his equal, he won't trust you.

Infecting His Sense of Trust:

♡ Befriend his competitors—the ones he hangs with, but you know competes with.

♡ Expect more generosity out of him. Like when out, look at the bill after he's paid and suggest he leave a bigger tip.

♡ Never compliment him or acknowledge his graciousness.

♡ Be quiet; this is shady to him. Act distant or too shy and you'll freak him out.

♡ Dislike children. Leo appreciates innocence and if you can't be down with that, you'll be on the outs with him.

Recognizing Motivation

Leo wants to conquer the world and has all the energy, wit, and charisma to get it done. No doubt Leo probably already has an army of people who stand behind him, preaching his name and motivating him onward. He's not to be messed with, because he's made of sheer determination. With an ego as big as the sun, Leo's got an invincible work ethic and is always out to prove something— how great, smart, charming, and successful he can be. No, getting him into action is never an issue; it's getting him to do what you wish that typically poses the problem.

Main cause
There's a lot of upkeep in being a megalomaniac.

Immunizing His Motivation

♡ Outshine him. Ask him to do something you know you're better at. Watch him then make a mockery of it instead. In the face of another person's victory, he'll lose his ability to be serious.

♡ Remove the spotlight. He wilts without it.

♡ If you don't want to go somewhere he prefers to, show up looking dowdy. He's so vain, he'll reconsider any place he might be seen with an unalluring date.

♡ Make him believe something he likes is outdated/uncool and it'll slowly make him lose interest.

♡ Get someone else to be the leader. Obeying makes him sleepy.

Infecting Him with Motivation:

♡ He's led by flattery. Always butter him up with a few well-placed compliments to get him to play into your requests. Two should do the trick.

♡ Ask him how to do something in order to get him to do it. There's nothing like letting Leo play the leader to get him into action.

♡ Make places sound exclusive and he won't be able to resist. He'll love anything expensive and elite sounding, as status drives his ego.

♡ He'll instantly like anyone if you tell him that person wants to meet him badly.

♡ Tell him he's vital to a plan. If Leo feels responsible for something, he'll take it all the way.

DESTINATION: DUMPSVILLE

Celestial Voodoo on You

It doesn't take an astrophysicist to figure out Leo's feelings are the only ones that matter. This can severely up his asshole factor when he's done with you. As a guy who's not into conflict, his common escape route is the disappearing act. His rule is that he answers to no one. If he wants to go off into the sunset, it's his prerogative and he doesn't have to claim any responsibility for anything other than his own happiness. If you happen to get caught up in his web and believed his fancy dialogue that had you thinking you were the only one and forever, then it'll suck to be you. With Leo, he is and will always be the only one. Not to say he didn't care, but things change and he can't be held responsible for how the future unravels, even if it's in a week or day that his feelings have flipped.

Sure, it's cold and unacceptable and if this is you, sorry. When it comes down to it, he doesn't give many warning signs. It could be one day he woke up and realized his feelings changed. Reasons can be anything, but it won't matter because once he's through, he's through, and you can rely on that. In his head, he justifies his behavior by focusing on the future, which is always a clean slate. It won't matter to Leo how he's left you unresolved or made you feel used. Also, with a dramatic and mysterious exit, it can sickly and egotistically leave you possibly wanting more—but don't fall for this twisted trap!

It's always best to realize how a man breaks up with you is a sign of his character and if Leo goes this route, know he's a dick and move on. If you chase after him, the only thing you're doing is validating his deluded ideas of grandeur. Yes, despite the fantastic whirlwind love affair he provided and all the magical things that he spewed from his mouth and was able to make you feel, cut your losses while you can. Leo coming back for an encore only spells trouble; he'll come back to screw out any respect he's left in you. You'll be left like a dirty rag that has been shredded of any good use when he's finished. In other words, don't let your suffering become his hard-on!

. . . And Other Signs He Hates You

The show must go on for Leo. If he hates you, he replaces you. No matter who you are, realize he always has a stand-in ready to take her mark alongside him. He makes it a point to have fans. If you no longer suit his needs and he has done all he could do with you, then down you go into the supporting-role ditch along with his other casualties. He reacts much like an animal that has taken a dump—he covers it up and moves on. He's a pro at coming out of a disaster with his hands clean, too. Even if he was the puppet master, he knows how to charm an audience and buy them if he has to. It's really pathetic if you think about it because it's just a superficial ploy to justify his false sense of superiority, but this is how he deals.

Of course, if there's a slight chance you have something that Leo still wants, don't expect for him to disappear yet. As long as you hold some kind of key for him, he won't burn his bridge. Instead, he'll slip into condescension mode and try to cover it with a smooth amount of charm. When he goes there, it should be pretty easy to figure it out (if you want to see it, that is). For lesser skilled Leos, give him time. His arrogant, vain, and utterly self-centered ways will eventually seep out because he'll feel too proud to need anyone. For the cleverer Leo, you can test his authenticity in two different ways. First, give him a compliment. If he doesn't seem flattered and takes it as a cue to go into a dialogue about himself, then yes, he's lost respect for your opinion and is using you. The other sign is if he gets cheap on you. If he makes both these foibles, then know you're officially on his shit list.

Beating Him to the Punch

However majestic Leo portrays himself, he can also be a big ole wimp. He'll howl like a banshee under the slightest discomfort, as he can't handle pain. The worst kind is the one that goes right to his ego, like being dumped. Know that no matter how you bid adieu, expect a scene.

With such a big head, getting rid of Leo requires sacrificing some of your own pride, as it's easier to get him to want to drive you away than to just dump him. As the dumped, he'll strive to save face. In addition, he has a charming way of getting himself out of trouble when he needs to. If you strike first, he'll try to sweet-talk his way back into your heart, and for unsuspecting individuals this can sometimes be shocking. It's as if he can change into another being instantly and be able to understand what you're feeling so well that you feel as if you have misjudged him. If he breaks this out, he's acting in order to win you back. Then, when you're safely in his clutches, he'll use his second chance to dump you, as he's competitive and needs to claim the last word.

If you mean business, dump him publicly and with a performance worthy of a standing ovation. This means being ready with the right outfit, scenery, and monologue. As long as you don't have an emotional breakdown and can control the scene, the humiliation will be too much for him to endure and he'll promptly take his cue to exit. If you need to jab deeper, have a new lover waiting in the wings ready to whisk you away from him. The degradation compounded with jealousy should beat him to an emotional pulp, which could only get more entertaining if Leo begins balling and crumbling to his knees. After all, drama feeds off drama. With such a sensational exit, this will win you a place in Leo's Breakup Hall of Fame, and a psychological platinum platter with the word WINNER monogrammed on it.

Ridding Yourself of Leo with Minimal Scarring:

- ♡ Publicly humiliate him.
- ♡ Be the star of the relationship by being the more outrageous and successful one.
- ♡ Have your own life with him as an obvious second. He likes people dependent on him, guaranteeing him the spotlight.
- ♡ Hate exhibitionism and repress his public image.
- ♡ Only want to go to quiet places that nobody frequents. Make your relationship super private.
- ♡ Stop caring about how you look in public and be a complete slob.
- ♡ Flirt with someone ugly and get caught.

Kick, Drop, and Kill

"What doesn't kill you makes you stronger" was probably first said by someone who just got out of a relationship with Leo. He's no messing around; he loves hard, plays hard, and ends it hard—hard for you, that is. Coming off of him is no easy task; it's like evacuating from a great party, complete with a gift bag upon exiting. However, instead of a material reward, what you get back is you. The fact is that you don't see the destruction until the fury of typhoon Leo has subsided, and assessing the aftermath can be a shock to the system. Things you'd never suspect you could have done are what you begin to see you did do—like forgo your own needs for him. Yes, he tends to suck up everything in his path and consume it for his own. Basically, the Leo experience is like a big wake-up call that leaves its victim asking what they want from themselves, how they really are living, and how they want to rebuild. In the end, along with great tales of romance and a splendid notch on your belt, you can take solace in the vital lesson Leo does teach: Always be the star of your own life and you can never go wrong.

WANTED: VIRGO

BORN: AUGUST 22—SEPTEMBER 22

Prissy know-it-all who communicates with condescension. Has a clean scent that can be tracked for miles. Possesses enviable bone structure and eyelashes, but he won't know what to do with them.

BARE BASICS

How to Spot Him

Virgo carries with him an air of aristocracy everywhere he goes. Along with his chiseled features and cleanly scrubbed attitude, he's always looking sophisticated and perfect for general consumption. It's as if he's man of the world, who's done, known, and seen it all. His cool expression would have strangers suspect he rarely sweats over much. Then, a drink spills on the floor and there he goes, nose-diving down to the ground, freaking out with paper towels in hand and an aggravated look that reeks of deadly intentions. In the world of Virgo, perfection can flip at the drop of a hat.

Yes, Virgo is a freakish man of distinction. He's all about portraying himself as flawlessly as possible, but in actuality he's a neurotic fiend who can't stop picking apart himself and the world around him. While he'll have an inconspicuous demeanor, it's a cover, allowing him a bird's-eye view of life to draw his conclusions—which are many. Although he'll say he's shy or will act it, he's not. The truth is he's got so many opinions it'd be too overwhelming to have them all spill out at once; so he retreats into politeness. Moderation is his way and his approach toward everything. When out in public, expect him to be cautiously blended into a crowd while maintaining his energy for something useful. Some days it's sulking, other days it's being a good citizen, and most other days are spent being an obsessive-compulsive germaphobe maniac in search of answers.

Yet, despite the insanity that's racing around in his brain, his heart is true. Virgo is not one to waste anything, least of all his affection. If you tickle his fancy, expect his spotlight to shine down upon you and be wowed with his impeccable manners and intelligent conversation. Being that he's so in tune with paranoia, the fabulous thing about him is that he offers himself wholly and free of mind games. His aim is to keep things as pure as they can be—and how he does it is with endless devotion. In other words, he's a complete sucker for love and there's nothing he won't do to get a piece of it, as it's the one thing that saves him from his cynicism. If he has found a possibility in you to get him to that promised land, where he'll be free from reason and the shackles of regimented living, then watch out. The fact of the matter is that the skeleton in Virgo's closet is that he's a die-hard romantic. If you happen to open the door to uncover this secret and feel intrigued, then it's best to walk in right away and shut that door quickly as he'd hate for his cover to be blown.

Key Features:

- ♡ Classic bone structure, high cheekbones, and long eye lashes
- ♡ A modest manner about him with a humble, yet somewhat condescending disposition
- ♡ A clean scent and appearance
- ♡ A busy energy that's nervous, yet reserved
- ♡ May have a tendency to have physical ticks of some sort

♡ Style that's thrifty, classic, or designer. He'll have clean lines, clean colors, and be perfectly arranged—as if he's coming from a photo shoot

♡ Highbrow conversationalist—researching everything so he can seem an expert

Seducing Him into Your Boudoir

If you're hot for him, you're going to have to spell it out. Virgo has a shaky sense of self that booms and wanes with confidence by the hour. His busy little mind produces manic thoughts by the second and his analyzing prowess churns away at top speed. If you catch his eye, his usual reaction is one of awkwardness. The contact will then set off a voice in his head that'll talk him in and out of every neurotic scenario as he's got a penchant for deconstructing anything he can wrap his brain around. Best to save the time, agony, and confusion by taking the reins.

Seizing control and showing that you like having it will be a huge turn-on for Virgo. This man loves to serve, and the best way for him to do his thing, with the maximum amount of efficiency, is by having specific orders. Not that being a bombastic fascist is going to lure him into your pants, but being direct will do the trick. He lives for perfection and organization; get him to come to you without adding any doubts in his mind. Once you have his attention, you're going to have to talk the talk, as the way into his heart is by stimulating his mind. It'll help if you're a part of MENSA (or pretend you are) because he thinks himself a highbrow intellectual and prefers to associate with the same. The fact is he has a bit of a snobby attitude, which is shocking considering how weaselly he can come across, but it's true. He has high goals for himself and longs for a brilliant lover with whom he can have involved conversations about life, beyond pop culture and other things of that petty nature. However, if you do happen to like Top 40 music, big budget movies, and tabloid magazines, don't be afraid. There's another surefire way to nail him—prove you've got status.

Yes, Virgos love dating up. If you've got a pedigree of any kind or any sort of impressive social quality or career, break it out, but without flaunting it. Drop the information in a subtle way and he'll pick it up. He pays attention to detail, so it's the little things you say that'll resonate the most with him. Despite his smarty-pant's attitude, the man is highly superficial and image is important. He'll forgo giving out his prerequisite IQ test for a chance at a ditzy member of a royal family, as having a sweetie with rank validates him and helps his insecurities. In fact, anything that can soothe his neurosis is a turn-on. Plus, being that he's naturally prone to being humble and modest, dating someone "higher up" means he'll have a guaranteed gold coin in his pocket to show off when he wishes. The bottom line is that he craves exclusiveness and if he sees you as a mentally stimulating VIP room, all he'll want to do is get inside. Of course, he's a gentleman through and through, and won't step in unless invited.

Loving Him in the Boudoir

Living to serve, aiming to please, and being endowed with an indomitable perfectionist attitude, you can count on Virgo to do you right. He's a worker bee, which means he's a hardworking lover who won't stop until everyone gets their pleasure. Just state your needs and reap the rewards. He's all about efficiency, too, so he'll stay focused at the matters at hand until he reaches success. Being a service-oriented man, expect to give Virgo a gold star every time he drops his drawers.

Make no mistake about his misleading symbol of the virgin, though, as he's pure in one sense and that is purely lethal. He's a horny bastard who loves sex as much as any sign. He just has a slightly different approach, as he's into being attuned to his physicality and working his muscles to ensure maximum performance. With sex, his one fault is that you might feel like exercise equipment at times, as he does a bit of cardio and weight training. But usually he needs approval so bad that he'll strive to see all your emotional needs are met too.

Plus, Virgo's a guy guaranteed to improve with practice. He loves learning, and when it comes to knowing your body, he'll want to study hard. He's the lover who'll pay attention to every little thing that turns you on and make mental notes. Of the talents he'll love perfecting the most: his oral, as he's the guy who loves, loves, loves to give it. So, make sure you've scrubbed really clean down there, because he'll be there for the long haul and has no problem going overtime—and the crazy thing is he's not doing it because he necessarily wants it back, but because he loves to give it. Now, how irresistible is that, being his all-you-can-eat smorgasbord without a price tag? Yes, it's quite obvious what makes Virgo a catch. Sexually, he's like having a free hooker at your beck and call and what kind of dummy would refuse that? Not one that he'd want to get involved with, that's for sure.

MAKING HIM COME TO THE PALM OF YOUR HAND

Eye Candy

Virgos like things uncomplicated. He likes clean lines, clean colors, and dry-clean-only labels on a squeaky clean lover. His aesthetic is easy and simple. For him, an effortless look is what's sexy—and this can mean a smart, casual no-frills style or chic fashion scooped up from the most underground part of some trendy locale. Practical and/or pristine looks are what he's drawn to. The naturalness of how you wear your clothes, not how they wear you, is what turns him on. Score bonus points with your overall upkeep, as refinement is Virgo's idea of picture perfection.

Stylin' Seduction:

- ♡ White. It's his color of choice.
- ♡ Modest style and solid colors that are fashionable, but never loud. It's all about subtlety with him.
- ♡ Dry-clean clothes only. Remember, he's about the finer things in life.
- ♡ Expensive fabrics, organic cottons, silk, etc. He pays attention to all the details—show you believe in good upkeep.
- ♡ Athletic and casual clothes that are comfy, but trendy. Function is as important as fashion.
- ♡ Good sneakers. Virgos have closets full of them.
- ♡ Labels, but only if they're subtle. He hates flashy names of designers on clothing. He thinks it's tacky when people are walking billboards.

Tasty Treats

Food

Turn the fussiness up with the ultimate finicky eater, because Virgo is the sign that's most prone to having dietary rules or food allergies of some type. Always find out his habits before booking reservations. Then, the next rule of thumb in feeding Virgo is nutrition. He's a health nut and typically sees food more as a functional need than a comfort zone. Not to say he's not into being wined and dined, but generally he eats with his body in mind and with the rare exception of indulgences on special occasions. To play it safe, though, stick to high-quality and high-performance foods to fuel your Virgo.

Erotic Eats:

- ♡ Gourmet restaurants. He likes to think he has distinguished tastes, to go with his whole highbrow persona. Even if he dislikes it, he'll have enjoyed the experience of trying something upscale.
- ♡ Restaurants with tasting menus. This way he can sample the chef's recommended specialties pre-set for him—no thinking in it! That sounds like fun already.
- ♡ Mexican. Haven't met a Virgo who doesn't like it.
- ♡ Vegetarian or vegan, or anything healthy. Load him up on the tofu (he'll need the protein for post-date activities).
- ♡ Experimental and modern foods. He's always into learning about new trends, as he wants to have an opinion on everything. Again, it won't matter if he hates the food, as long as he'll gain a new opinion when he's done.
- ♡ His regular haunts. Virgos love their routines.
- ♡ Food made at the table, like hibachi. He loves seeing the process of things being made.

Movies

Virgo lives for perfection. It's his lifetime goal. In having such an unattainable aspiration, it allows him to constantly indulge his favorite activity—thinking. He loves thinking about anything and everything because being perfect means having all the answers. So, realize everything he does revolves around this addiction. If you do need to intervene, take him to a silly and frivolous mainstream movie so he can escape his thoughts. If anything, make fun of its trivialness—but only if your Virgo happens to have a sense of humor. If you've got an analyzing junkie who can't go a few hours without a dose of purpose, then get your tickets early for flicks with depth and something complex in its message or plot. Otherwise he'll consider it a torture to have sit in the dark and be "dumbed" down.

Cinematic Foreplay:

- ♡ Mystery/suspense. He'll clock how long it takes for him to figure it out before everyone else.
- ♡ Foreign films. Subtitled movies are always good, as he assumes they're more intellectual.
- ♡ Movies with animals. He's a sucker for all the world's other creatures.
- ♡ Documentaries or anything educational is superb. He's always up for learning!
- ♡ Black comedy. Nothing beats a good evil laugh.
- ♡ Coming-of-age dramas. He'll relate, he's always coming into himself.
- ♡ Indie flicks that everyone is talking about, and anything else he can critique with others.

Dating Ideas

As the original Mr. Pleaser, Virgo will probably be insistent in doing what you want and adapt to your needs right away. For him, it's more of a kick to get to know you, how you function and how you can fit into his life. However, if you want to avoid being the one under examination, suggest situations where you can really see what's he's about—places that are part of his routine, as his life is built upon habits. Watch him in his natural habitat and get your best data. Of course, if you want to fast-forward and step it up, bring him to a place where there's competition, as his selfless guise will fade fast and you can really see what he's got up there in his ego. Yes, behind his passiveness is a heart of a fighter.

Playful Planning:

♡ Sporting events, but less mainstream sports. He's not the regular football and baseball type. Go for tennis, lacrosse, soccer, etc. Anything deemed more highbrow is more his speed.

♡ Hiking or any sort of nature adventure. If animals can be integrated into this, even better.

♡ Museums, botanical gardens. Anything cultural is good. He's always up for brain food.

♡ A lecture or anything of that intellectual caliber.

♡ An arcade or mini-golf. He's highly competitive and you can see it emerge best in low energy games.

♡ A car dealership. Take him to test cars; he'll love vicariously living through sampling.

♡ Factory tours. He loves seeing how things are made.

Sound Seduction

Conversation

Virgo loves to communicate, but not just to babble. facts randomly, go on about himself, or any sort of irrelevance. This is the guy who wants to have a point and get to it. He likes conversations with purpose. He's keen on intellectual matters, loves to discuss facts, and appreciates debates as a place to share his knowledge and theories. While he may be humble about many things, his mind is the one thing he'll boast about, and he usually thinks he's the smartest person in the room. Challenge him for the title and impress him to no end.

Icebreakers:

♡ Engage him in a conversation about politics. He's always up for debates on that. Warning, he may play devil's advocate just to keep you going.

♡ Discuss ideas of what makes up a perfect society. Get him to describe it: the people in it, the government, etc. Anything that deals with perfection, he'll have an opinion on how to achieve it.

♡ Ask him for career advice. He loves dishing about work and offering his opinions on such matters.

♡ Ask about his most psycho love story. You'll learn another side to him that you won't readily suspect.

♡ Ask for his first impression of you and get his psychological analysis of you. He forms an immediate profile on everyone he meets.

♡ Describe his perfect day. This'll give you more personal facts.

♡ Get him to give critiques on movies, music, performers, etc. Better yet, ask him his opinion on something you suspect he'd loath—like a vapid pop-culture blockbuster movie. He loves complaining, but prepare to hear more than your fair share of negative comments.

Music

Think of Virgo like a satellite, in the know with everything. Although he won't like everything he's tuning into, he'll be aware of it. This makes him open to everything, as he'll want to have an opinion to say "yay" or "nay." As for what he'll actually admit to liking, this will depend on the crowd he runs with—as many have totally cornball tastes that bring shame. Seeing that he's trying to come across so cool, his admitted music tastes will be hipper than thou. Beyond the peer-pressure aspect, though, he'll generally gravitate toward music of musicians: mind-expanding sounds that have an experimental element, smartness, or a completely raw/organic feel to it. If it's angry, he'll also go for that—it gives him an avenue for release, an action that he's always into.

Mood Makers:

- ♡ Psychedelic rock. Mind altering music appeals to him.
- ♡ Irreverent music, random things like TV show tunes and stuff like that. Indulge his quirky side.
- ♡ Electronica. Music that is modern and made with technology is his thing.
- ♡ Classical. Soothing brain music can never go wrong with him.
- ♡ Songs with smart lyrics. He's all for music that songwriters would respect, as he likes anything "smart."
- ♡ Avant-garde/minimalist. Anything experimental is his speed.
- ♡ Angry-sounding music—metal: death, speed, or heavy. Hard-core punk. Gangsta rap. It helps relieve his tensions.

Gifts

Mr. Virgo is 99 percent practicality, 1 percent excess—as far as the material. He's not typically a guy to get caught up with clutter, unless it's papers, like periodicals, but that's another story. As for objects he holds near and dear, there'll be few. He's a guy who likes function, and everything he owns has a use. Even though gifts are meant to have a sense of extravagance, don't do him the favor of treating him to something luxurious if it's not practical in some way. For example, sure get him that Gucci watch, but avoid the Gucci license plate frame. Understand?

Boxed Treats:

- ♡ Gift certificates to Internet music download sites. Non-physical clutter is good.
- ♡ Electronic portable gadgets. Anything that maximizes efficiency.

♡ Clothes with a cool label please, but remember nothing ostentatious. Designer names must be subtle or strictly on the inside only.

♡ Tickets to a sporting event. Any excuse to yell is his idea of a good time.

♡ Bath products or cleaning products. A Dirt Devil would be deemed a romantic present.

♡ Video games or accessories for play. He's all about technology as entertainment.

♡ Exercise-related items. He's the sign of fitness.

Touch Me

Don't underestimate Virgo's sexual prowess by his reserved demeanor because you'll be short-changing yourself of a hot and furious piece of sexual dynamite ready to detonate in your pants at your request. The fact is this guy gives Deluxe Sex. He's not in it just for the physical sensation, but out to learn something deeper about himself, you, and life itself. Sure, some of the lesser evolved Virgos who are wired just for efficiency are purely in it for the release, but for the most part, the typical Virgo is an earthy lover that views sex as a vital bodily function that can transport the mind to a higher plane. He yearns to explore all the mechanics of sex and with someone of the same mind-set.

In getting the most out of your Virgo, you must mentally tantalize him. The more your brilliance tickles his curiosity, the more you prove your capacity to excite him in the right places. Things like being able to keep up with his cynical jokes and outlandish intellectual jabber are the fuel he'll need to see where and how far you go with him. He wants to see your hunger for knowledge, as that's what he considers sexy and drives him mad. So, break out your manifestos and keep his mind enthralled. Once the lights turn off, he'll barely be able to keep himself from ravishing you.

To bring him over the top, share your appreciation for his sexual abilities; that's what keeps him driven in the sack. Virgo is a man who needs reassurance, and with sex, it'll be more necessary. There are so many voices in his head; he needs to know which one to listen to—so make yours stand out with a positive message. Scream it loud and proud, make him hear, smell, touch, taste, and see your enthusiasm. Boost him higher and higher into a sex-god state. Then reap those rewards, as your body becomes his ambrosia. Virgo is so stimulated by pleasuring his lovers that it has been reported that he has the ability to come from just hearing his lover come—and this includes not even touching himself in any way. Now how incredible is that?

The fact is, he's a sensitive guy who approaches sex like a mutual language, and the clearer you are in your demands, the more specific Virgo will be in fulfilling his manly duties. The more he can get you off, the hotter he becomes and the more poetic your creation. The deal with Virgo is the more you appreciate what he puts out, the more he'll put into you.

Ways to Heat Up Your Virgo:

- ♡ Lie next to him and stroke his stomach area lightly with your fingertips. Tease his erogenous zone. Also, start a conversation on anything he'd deem "intellectual." You're now stroking his favorite organ, his mind.
- ♡ Do him after a shower and don't forget to have clean sheets with a laundry-fresh scent. This will add to his comfort and his performance.
- ♡ Be verbally explicit. The more direct your demands, the better his drive.
- ♡ Be loud in bed and moan hard. He gets off on hearing how good he is.
- ♡ Wear virginal lingerie. Purity is romantic.

- ♡ Tease him with sexy text messages, e-mails, or whatever you've got to communicate your lust.
- ♡ Surprise him with a blow job while he's surfing the Net. He'll love the raunchy research multitasking.

Role-playing

Anything that involves planning turns Virgo on. In the sexual theater arena, he'll take it as serious as an opening night on Broadway. He'll start as head of pre-production, ensuring you the best in costumes, props, setting, and even the ever so vital lighting. No doubt, he'll go all out to make the stage set for maximum play. The characters he'd easily be inclined to get off in will be ones that are subordinate in some way or have some sort of massive responsibility to himself or the greater good of mankind. If this will mean getting his ass beat a little, then that's going to have to be.

Cast of Characters:

- ♡ Lab animal and scientist. Transform your boudoir into a lab and have the lab animal get loose and sexually assault the scientist. This will appeal to his inner smutty researcher.
- ♡ Future versions of yourselves in an alternate world. He's got a sci-fi thing in him.
- ♡ Dean and a naughty professor in need of tenure. Academia turns him on.
- ♡ Shrink and sexual addict patient. Analysis is his thing.
- ♡ Carnival freak and circus ringmaster. They all think they're freaks.
- ♡ Celebrities of choice. Make it random; put famous names in a hat and then pick it out. Don't tell the other who you're playing and surprise each other.
- ♡ Fantasy characters, like Godzilla and Mothra or dirty Smurfs. It allows him to use his imagination, but with a reference point—which will be more comfortable for him.

Taking the Bait

Virgo loves to fall in love, because being in love equals obsession and obsession means lots of work to be done. In this state, Virgo has the perfect reason to go on a research binge. Yes, within every Virgo is the propensity to be a maniac groupie, wanting to know every detail of their subject's existence—and that means any random connection, too. This will include anything and everything that may vaguely be attached to you, down to researching all your hobbies, career, the company you work for, your culture, the town where you grew up, the college you attended, music you like, the car you drive, your astrological makeup—everything! No subject is off limits and anything that's remotely associated with you is a morsel of gold.

He won't be obvious with all his detective work, as Virgo hates to be seen as vulnerable. However, the info will be dropped out during conversations as random facts he just happens to know. Go ahead and test it out. Bring up a vacation you took to some remote area and in a week bring the subject up again. Miraculously, he'll suddenly be able to tell you the population of the area, their bird, and the local cuisine's secret spice. The more bizarre the tidbits of info, the deeper his crush is on you.

With everything, Virgo is after the facts. He'll strive to know who you are and what makes you tick. After all, before he gets involved with anything, he has to know what he's heading into. To ensure his safety, he'll create his psychological report, cross-referencing your information with his to make a proper analysis of your relationship's nucleus, direction, and potential. Plus, this is his way of grasping all your dimensions, which will then help him do the best job in serving you—making his offer of sexy companionship perfect and irresistible, as he loves with the passion of a fanatic, minus the creepiness.

UNAUTHORIZED: ASTRAL AUTOPSY

Recognizing Fear

The life of a Virgo runs on rails. He has schedules to keep and goals to meet. Yes, he's a control freak and if anything deviates from his preconceived plans, expect havoc. When left without a reference point, he'll feel clueless, confused, scared, and ultimately in a claustrophobic state of uncertainly.

Main cause
The inevitability of the unexpected.

Immunizing His Fears:

♡ Always have Internet access ready to research at a moment's notice, and have all your gadgets charged to full power.

♡ Get a routine down with him. Virgo thrives with schedules.

♡ If you have a high IQ, let him know. He'll feel safer the higher your points are.

♡ Clip coupons. Extravagance makes him nervous. Be a cautious spender, unless it's to promote yours/his vanity.

♡ Articulateness is a prerequisite for his lovers. Be aware of the details to everything. When making plans, give definitive time frames, addresses, description of locales, etc.

Infecting Him with Fear:

♡ Don't inform him of plans you have until the last minute.

♡ When going somewhere new, leave the maps and directions at home (meanwhile, you should memorize how to get there) and inform him of this foible thirty minutes into your trip.

♡ Have him deal with anything unhygienic. To really upset him, "accidentally" sneeze on him right before his vacation or weekend.

♡ Don't fill up the gas tank until the red light turns on.

♡ Take him out to clubs or parties where he'll think he's not cool enough. This will mean any place that's clean with well-dressed patrons.

Recognizing Anger

Virgo is a total hothead. He's got a quick temper, and little things piss him off. He loves his routines and has peculiar habits. Mess with his methods, mess with his mind, and answer to his wrath. He lives with the idea that perfection can exist, striving for it every day. Obviously, unless he lives in a box without any stimulus, imperfection is unavoidable—which means so is his anger. Plus, to escalate his anger, he takes it all quite personally, making these situations even more ridiculous.

Main cause
Living in an imperfect world.

Immunizing His Anger:

♡ Be on time and stick to your word. Be perfect.

♡ Be anal and be aware of everything. For example, if you pick out something of his to look at, put it back exactly where you found it.

♡ Never tell him he's crazy. All Virgos think they should be locked up and fear being institutionalized.

♡ Be as efficient as possible, like always make sure you get on the shortest lines and find the closest parking spaces.

♡ Be a worrywart. Having to deal with your neurosis will divert his own.

Infecting Him with Anger:

- ♡ Beat him at Scrabble, Chess, Trivial Pursuit, or any game where his intelligence is on the line.
- ♡ Never clean the hair out of the shower drain or leave garbage, like used ketchup packets, in his car—anything deemed dirty will bug him.
- ♡ Use too much toilet paper or forget to replace the roll when empty. Wastefulness and inefficiency make him burn.
- ♡ Speak with improper grammar.
- ♡ Be late with movie rentals and subject him to pay the fee. You'll never have to return a video after you mess up once.

Recognizing Sadness

Existential agony is a constant struggle most Virgos must attend to. Being such a thorough thinker, it would be impossible for him not to fall under his own scrutiny and of what he perceives is others' judgments. With constant analysis going on, a veil of sadness is perpetually covering Virgo's mind. His reality is that he must take on the weight of the world and feel bad for the vicious cycle that we call life.

Main cause
Life is sad.

Immunizing His Sadness:

- ♡ Always ask him about work; it's vital that he's productive and gets acknowledged for it.
- ♡ Quote him to others and have him "accidentally" overhear. The ego boost will make him happy into the next lifetime.
- ♡ Smell clean all the time. A laundry-fresh scent is like a stress-reducing aromatherapy candle.

♡ Call him up to fix stuff around your house or with your computer. Keep a long to-do list, as keeping him busy and needing him is a factor in his upkeep.

♡ Talk crap about people he hates with him. Nothing like putting down others as a social activity to keep him in good spirits.

Infecting Him with Sorrow:

♡ Upset him with germs. Double dip into the salsa or touch his face after using public transportation.

♡ React to his style with a giggle and a look of compassion — but tell him he looks good. He's super-delicate about his appearance, and any slight undermining will cause a silent pity party.

♡ Bring up a story expressing how smart you think a close friend or coworker is, but also make your examples fairly unimpressive. Not only will he get sad having you think anyone else but him is a genius, he'll also be upset thinking you actually have low standards for intelligence.

♡ Never remember his routines or his "regulars," like his favorite drink or dinner at a particular restaurant. If you don't pay attention to his details, he'll think you don't know him.

♡ Put on a sad movie that deals with an animal. He has endless compassion for all living creatures, except the human.

Recognizing Trust

For Virgo, trust isn't just being able to lend you $50 and get it back the next day. No, it's his ability to trust your judgments, and that means your intelligence and morality. While loyalty and honesty may be a part of it, too, it weighs far less than your deductive reasoning skills. He gauges your smarts by studying how well you understand him, follow his thought process, and if you can agree with it. If you pass his tests, you're then deemed bright enough to recognize genius and therefore able to be confided in by one.

Main cause
Only intelligent people deserve value.

Immunizing His Trust:

♡ If you have a degree from a highly accredited university and/or high SAT scores, subtly drop that info. If you're too blatant with this info, he'll think you're bragging—and he'll be turned off by your boastful behavior. By knowing this tidbit of info, it'll prove you're smart in the traditional sense and in turn prove your worthiness for his trust.

♡ Know and use big words properly and naturally.

♡ Always clean anything you borrow from him and return promptly.

♡ Squeeze the toothpaste from the bottom up and put the cap back when done. He's more trusting of people who pay attention to details like these.

♡ Be a germaphobe. This will show you're on his wavelength.

Infecting His Sense of Trust:

♡ Lose your keys once or misplace your wallet. He'll consider this a permanent reflection of your lack of awareness.

♡ Have an old operating system in your computer and he'll think you're outdated and an unreliable source for information.

♡ Talk in generalities; he'll consider this evasive behavior and instantly get suspicious. He's a total neurotic.

♡ Go places with him and run short on cash, needing him to pick up your slack. Anywhere he is needed, he'll kindly adhere to, as he lives to serve—but not with this wallet. Money is how he gauges power.

♡ Pull a practical joke during a serious moment. For example, if you're going to the airport, pretend you left your passport at home. Cry wolf with him once and that's it.

Recognizing Motivation

If there's a point A and a point B, you'll find Virgo on its most direct path. He hates aimlessness and lives for results. He rarely does anything without a reason, loving efficiency and productivity. This may lead him to get lazy if he finds no goal to aim for or a way to keep himself constantly occupied (but this will depend on the genetics of your Virgo in question, too). Either way, to get him to operate properly, think of a factory and how it's run, then apply it to him.

Main cause
Results are necessary in getting his ass in gear.

Immunizing His Motivation:

♡ Bring him into dirty and germ-invested environments. Nothing closes him up quicker than being in an unsavory space.

♡ Cry and create emotional turmoil. Feelings scare him, especially intense ones. He deals best with facts.

♡ Don't set deadlines, as he can't function without structure.

♡ Bring him somewhere he must be happy, easygoing, and accepting. He won't know what to do, but shut down.

♡ He picks up hints easily. If you ask him to do something with less than excited enthusiasm, you can count him out. He's all about the reassurance.

Infecting Him with Motivation:

♡ Be unorganized when doing some kind of manual chore you don't want to do. Your poor skills will frustrate him and force him to save you with his efficiency prowess. For example, if you have to assemble a piece of furniture (although he lives to do Mr. Fix It things like this), fumble about and do it haphazardly. At the end, his love of being useful will outweigh his aggravation at you.

♡ Have a task that involves proving who's the smartest. This will move him into action fast.

♡ He loves bargains, no matter what they are. Whatever you want or wherever you want to go, make it seem inexpensive or pay for him. He does anything if it's complimentary.

♡ Anything that requires a lot of detail and patience calls for Virgo. Projects that require precision—he's your man.

♡ Need information. Research is his inspiration—he lives for digging any facts, cross-referencing prices, and things of that nature.

DESTINATION: DUMPSVILLE

Celestial Voodoo on You

Virgo has three main routes he goes to end a relationship: first, being his usual practical self and dumping you straight on with facts and logic, second, fading you from his routines slowly. The third is the worst, when he needs to seek revenge. In this case, Virgo can turn into one sick motherfucker who will plot out your demise with the precision of a brain surgeon and the maliciousness of a middle school bully. He's got no qualms screwing with your life, starting with pushing psychological buttons. Yes, in picking up the details to pleasure you, he's also picked up the little things that irk you. With that information, he'll take great joy to jab you in the most vulnerable spots of your psyche. Don't resist his sadistic ways or fight with him, as this then challenges him to a battle of wills. If he has it in him, he can be stubborn and will hold out to destroy you, because his insecurity drives him to be highly competitive.

If you confront him, he'll deny it by talking his way through the situation and having you wonder if you're going nuts. He'll strike you in your psyche and If you aren't clever to figure out his methods, then you might be in for a disastrous ride to Crazyville. To Virgo, screwing with your mind is a form of fun, because it proves how smart he is—and he can never get enough of proving that to himself. In the end, he needs to be thorough, as he is about everything, and that means destroying any shred of happiness that he can receive from you. Not like he means to be so sadistic, but he can't help turning into a mad scientist when making an attempt at love. If the experiment went bad and he can't explain it, the only thing left to do is to dissect it. Unfortunately for you, if he cuts too deep, oh well. Sometimes people have to get hurt in perfecting his ideals.

. . . And Other Signs He Hates You

Virgo has a super nasty side that comes out when he no longer needs your approval. This means playing with your head for fun, like a cat dangling a mouse before the kill. However, Virgo won't kill; he'll keep you on the brink of life and wishing you were dead. Plus, he's slick, so the signs will be subtle. The most evident will be his condescension, as he'll have a way of making you feel dumb and undermine your confidence. To add to your misery, he's also into sabotage. Avoid asking advice from him if you suspect he's got any animosity toward you. If he hates you, then he'll give you misleading information that is meant to screw with you. All the while, he'll be getting off on watching you scamper about. This then proves how gullible you are and how brilliant he is. With this, he'll think himself like an all-knowing god, being able to control you as he wishes. Just realize though, this sadist side only comes out in the face of pure disgust—the disgust against his own poor judgment. In hating himself, he'll take it out on you and punish you for reminding him that he can't be perfect.

Beating Him to the Punch

He prides himself on being efficient, and when being dumped you'd only hope he'd follow suit. If not, expect Virgo's automatic reaction to be Mr. Fix It mode. He won't even question his own happiness in the relationship, as his instincts are driven to correct the wrongs, even if there are none. So, come prepared when dumping Virgo; have pie charts, exact dates, or any hard evidence to prove your case. His defense will be working it like a debate club meeting, aiming for you to take all the blame as he strives to keep himself immaculate of fault. Keep tight on the reins, though, and make the situation like you're the boss firing him as the employee. If this makes you the bad guy, realize it's a small price to pay.

With Virgo, there's never an easy way to put it; he's so bent on being perfect that when faced with something as conceptual as a breakup, it makes it hard for him to deal. Most of the time, his issues won't even be about you, but with his own insanities about failure and being right. So, keep this in mind and refrain from getting sucked into his madness. Ignore his possible taunting and the low blows he might pull. If he goes there, tune him out. The trick is to make him feel stupid because that's how he'll slink away. Otherwise, he'll look to create a never-ending knot of psychological twister, giving you a chronic case of Virgo. The antidote: Realize how ridiculous he is and leave it at that. Yes, making him feel like a moron is your cure.

Ridding Yourself of Virgo with Minimal Scarring:

♡ Speak in slang in public. Use words improperly and grammatically incorrect.

♡ Get super lazy and unmotivated. He abhors the unproductive.
♡ Hate his pets.
♡ Waste money.
♡ Only see black and white, forget the gray in between. They are irrelevant to you—essential to him.
♡ Be flashy and put him under the spotlight often.
♡ Ignore planning and prefer to play things by ear.

Kick, Drop, and Kill

Virgos like to teach and once you graduate from his austere institution, you're guaranteed to come out wiser. Even if it's just learning that you'll never date a Virgo again, practical knowledge is a gift he bestows to his lovers. However, chances are the wisdom he grants is of greater self-awareness, as he's criticized, penalized, deconstructed, and reconstructed you so many times that it'd be impossible for you to avoid your own self-examination. This can leave you new and improved or drained and maimed. Either way, you'll come out with a deeper understanding of what makes you human and gives you character.

Assuming you didn't let Virgo's persnickety behavior get the better of you, leaving him behind gives you back your space to breathe and appreciate your imperfections (and the world's). In time your sense of humor will return, and most important, laughing will no longer seem like a judgment. Then, when the dust settles and Virgo looks back to sneer at you, which is 99 percent certain, your renewed self will most likely shake his delicate senses, giving him something to think about. Ultimately, it'll be a win-win situation for everyone and what could be more perfect than that?

WANTED: LIBRA

BORN: SEPTEMBER 23–OCTOBER 22

 Attractive charmer with an effectively evasive way of conversing. Tends to be fashionably styled and highly creative; responsibility and punctuality not included. Will attach to your hip easily.

BARE BASICS

How to Spot Him

One look at him and you can feel your heart throbbing faster, as if Cupid has shot an arrow right into you—and it's not just because he's so beautiful. With Libra, there's something more, something beyond skin deep. Although it would be easy to get intimidated by his leading-man good looks, which cast an awe-inspiring presence that oozes charm and refinement, he'll surprise you with his modesty, making him just that much more devastatingly gorgeous. Like a magnificent piece of art, rare is there a soul immune to his magnetism, and with more time spent in his company, the more he'll envelop you. Yes, with every flash of his dazzling smile, expect to lose a bit of your self-control.

To say the least, Libra isn't the guy who has any trouble getting laid. However, the precious fact about him is that he's no slut. While he loves sex and all the attention being a wildly handsome creature brings him, he's a traditionalist at heart and would rather have one true love than a million worshippers. For him, partnerships make him thrive, and despite his flirty ways, he likes having one person on whom to focus his attention. With that soul mate lover of his, he'll unlock his serious side and his highest potentials. By being able to balance himself with another, he can have the reassurance and validation he needs to feel invincible.

In the meantime, while looking for the one to love, he'll saunter about town, indulging in as many scenes as possible. Typically being artistically gifted, Libra can usually be found at the coolest of the cool places and hob-knobbing with an elite crowd. Not that he gets too caught up in the snobbery, he just likes pretty ambiances with a creative feel. To Libra, having stylish attire and a perfectly coiffed appearance is just part of the fun and another way to express himself, as he's not a guy that takes himself too seriously. He likes to be dressed for any opportunity that can arise, as more times than not, how his day begins can often be the opposite of how it ends.

Not one to plan far in advance, Libra prefers to take life and love as it comes. While he's a romantic at heart and can fall in love at first sight, he doesn't like losing his decorum and will be somewhat reserved when initially sharing his feelings. Smooth with his introductions, Libra can make it hard to decipher whether he wants to fuck you or be friends, but that's just his way. He doesn't like coming on strong or phony, and he wants to give you space to show who you are. All the while, he'll be taking you in as if he's sampling a fine wine. He'll check out the label, smell the aromas, swish the body about, then slowly sip in the flavor and see how the taste settles. As he cleanses his palette to see if he desires more, he'll progress accordingly. Being a patient and graceful gentleman, he likes taking his time in staking his claim—as rushing is never his style. Luckily for you, he's so hot that just staring at him while he casually falls in love with you should be just fine.

Key Features:

- ♡ A symmetrical face, classic good looks, and a picture-perfect smile
- ♡ A debonair air about him — a gentleman's demeanor
- ♡ Stylish and trendy looking—found in hip places
- ♡ A soft-spoken voice
- ♡ Hanging with a crowd and usually a fashionable crowd in an attractive place
- ♡ Has an artistic nature
- ♡ Generous to a fault (this could also be to his detriment, as many a Libra are bad with budgets)

Seducing Him into Your Boudoir

Rule #1: If a Libra raises your brow, make sure he's single. Finding a lone Libra is a rare occurrence, like witnessing the Abominable Snowman. If he's truly unattached, best to double-check. The logic is that since partnerships are his forte, a bachelor Libra can be a red flag unto itself. In many cases it can be a tip-off to any number of issues that are invisible to the naked eye, such as extreme possessiveness, skilled con artistry, or a tiny dick. Typically, the only datable Libras are the ones who have been safely out of a relationship for at least three weeks and have had a healthy number of them under his belt.

Sure, it's not the most romantic way to start a seduction, but if you can be smooth about it, then half your battle has already been won, because showing off your casual cool will nab his attention. Plus, by confirming his status you have also unwittingly charmed him by fearlessly taking the lead—and nothing makes Libra hotter than knowing he's being hunted like a piece of meat. That's right, forget trying to wow him with your sweetness or how you love your family or showing off your genius IQ, even if you're in the midst of curing cancer.

While all those attributes are wonderful, what really gets him to swoon will be revealing how dazzled you are by his looks. Comments acknowledging his style, his hair, and of course, his coolness factor will do the trick, but of course, you must be able to hold your own in these categories to make your compliments a trusted judgment. Treat picking him up like buying a piece of art: Judge for aesthetics and be respectful toward its intrinsic value.

Then, after you make your lusty intentions known, you'll have to slow it down. While Libra might like you to be a bit forward to jump-start the courtship, he'll be turned off by aggressive behavior if it continues. He's a mellow guy and prefers the naturalness of attraction to unravel at its own pace. While you can nudge the speed along, jumping the gun is never a good idea, as he equates pushiness with being déclassé. The lovers he looks to bed are ones with social graces that can blend with royalty if need be. Of course, when all is said and done, once those doors shut, break out your high-class hooker moves and let him know what's outside is only a taste of the real treasure on the inside.

Loving Him in the Boudoir

Libra pursues his lusts like a main character in an epic romance, striving to make each conquest worthy of being a chapter in his ravishing collection of love stories that would warm even the coldest heart. To him, sex is not a raunchy sweat fest that's pleasing to the body and at times the mind—that would be too common. Sex is about the soul, an expression of its passion, and a way to intensely connect with another. Orgasm is then the culmination of that experience, the finale to the creation of a beautiful moment. Idealistic, yes. Impossible, never. He's an optimist and romantic through and through and believes in this potential for every sexual exchange he finds himself in.

So, forget the sleazy and self-satisfying appeal to fucking and the casual feel to screwing; with Libra it's about making love—skilled, sensual, and graceful body-rolling love. In this approach, you'll be pleased to find he won't just focus on one aspect of the sex, but rather the complete process—meaning tender pre and post coitus moments. His aim is to have your souls touch and as sweetly as possible. To ensure this happens, he'll go to great lengths to be aware of your needs and adjust himself accordingly to blend your energies together for maximum pleasure. Plus, he won't skimp on the details, as it's those final touches that can make these memories last forever. Particulars such as the lighting, music, elixirs, incense, costumes, and any other accoutrements reeking of romance turn him on. Libra understands the more that comes out of him, then the more that'll come out of you.

MAKING HIM COME TO THE PALM OF YOUR HAND

Eye Candy

If you want to run with Libra's crowd, you better know how to dress— and we're not just talking color coordination. With Libra you have to step it up and show you have an acute eye for style, as if you're the premier fashion editor to the universe. As the ultimate clotheshorse, Libra won't even entertain the thought of being with anyone who doesn't present well. Dress like you're about to strut down a runway to capture his imagination, but also note he's a "we" not "me" thinker, and looking good as a couple will be a major consideration for him. So, do your part and dress like half of a visual masterpiece, and of course, top it all off with blue-blood social graces and he'll be wrapped around your finger in no time.

Stylin' Seduction:

- ♡ Royal blue, pink, and green colors. Pull them off and turn him on.
- ♡ Good hair. It's always good to have at least one hair product around him.
- ♡ Classic looks. No raunchy clothing, please. Even to go to bed, be ready to look cute 24-7.
- ♡ Well-fitted and tailored outfits that play up your sexuality a touch, but not overtly. He likes modesty, but with flair.
- ♡ Hip labels. It's about being cool with this one.
- ♡ Different looks and styles. He appreciates someone that isn't a one-trick fashion pony.
- ♡ Great accessories. Topping looks off with added touches is a trait only a real style maven can pull off. Note: Good sunglasses are a prerequisite to a good wardrobe.

Tasty Treats

Food

Libra was born to live the high life and undoubtedly, his tastes are expensive. Whether this is put on, acquired, or really natural can be anyone's guess, but his palate tends to crave flavors that are delicate, highbrow, and/or stylish. However, good food is only half the requirements of a good Libran dining experience, as good company and ambiance are equal in importance. To ensure him a fabulous time, he needs first-rate service and atmosphere down to the last detail: from the music, decor, wine list, views, to the menu's design. All in all, to score points with him, think beyond nutritional requirements.

Erotic Eats:

- ♡ Sushi, the perpetual hipster favorite. Plus, he prefers light foods and things that won't make him feel bloated.
- ♡ Fine dining. Places with a dress code and valet parking appeal to his sense of sophistication.
- ♡ The newest restaurant. Any place that has the trendy foods, a hot crowd, and stylish music will appeal to Libra.
- ♡ A restaurant with a good wine list. He's a connoisseur of all things sophisticated.
- ♡ Bistros. You can never go wrong with a traditional romantic kind of ambiance.
- ♡ Caviar and champagne locales. The more exclusive, the better.
- ♡ Alfresco dining with a casual vibe. Places that let diners linger. Libra is all about bonding in nature.

Movies

Ruled by Venus, Libra is the sign in charge of the arts, making him a complete snob when it comes to cinema. So, forget frivolous films with an entertainment value set at the lowest common denominator. He won't have that. Libra needs movies with merit, by serious directors with a strong vision, actors that believe their work is a craft, beautiful visuals, spectacular costumes, an incredible soundtrack, and an intelligent script. Think films worthy of respectable festivals and you'll hit the spot; he'd rather eat dirt than waste time with trash. Think pretentiously and you're getting the idea.

Cinematic Foreplay:

- ♡ Foreign flicks. It's always a smart choice, because it's cool, hip, and artsy.

♡ Arthouse/indie movies. Films that aren't made by sell-outs are his speed.

♡ Cinematic masterpieces that have epic cinematography, like Peter Greenaway films. Pretty works with him.

♡ Romance. All Libras are lovers.

♡ Courtroom drama or any films dealing with justice and over-coming evil. He's the sign of harmony.

♡ Award-winning movies, festival winners. These are officially highbrow enough for him.

♡ Documentaries on artistic genuis mesmerize him.

Dating Ideas

As long as he's got company, Libra is fine. Plus, being an adaptable kind of guy, he's always open to suggestions. The only non-debatable aspect is the pace he likes to move at, which is always leisurely. He hates having to rush. This makes activities that are more of the mind and less of the body suited toward his comfort. Not to say he's lazy, as he's usually on the go, but he likes to keep situations smooth and mellow. Cultural pursuits or chill social atmospheres tend to be the best places for him, since he likes getting transported into environ-ments that he can feed off and pleasantly blend with.

Playful Planning:

♡ Parties. He'll have no problem hitting the town and checking out your scene. Plus, he'll like checking out the social merger that may go on between the two of you as a couple.

♡ Museums, art openings, and theater. Artsy stuff is always cool with Libra.

♡ Live music events. The more underground, the better.

♡ A sunset date where you meet up to share a bottle of wine to take in the view. Libra loves this sort of serene romance.

♡ Clubbing and dancing. He's great at tripping the light fantastic.
♡ Peace rally or some form of justice-seeking event. He's all into defending what's right.
♡ A hike, bike ride, or slow stroll through a nice park, especially one with a dog run. Libra is a dog's best friend.

Sound Seduction

Conversation

Libras are fabulous conversationalists. He has an elegant way of speaking and knows just enough to carry on delight banter about anything—being that he was born to perform well at cocktail parties. Also, as the ruler of the arts and harmony, and being an air sign, discussions that lean away from the personal and more about culture and/or current affairs are up his alley. He'll like bonding with others over common tastes, such as music, film, art, fashion, and travel. Think arts and leisure section of the paper and your words are sure to be a page-turner.

Icebreakers:

♡ Ask him about which artists he admires. This will give you insight into who he aspires to be.
♡ Talk about love; ask him to define it. He'll score major points, as he's got the tongue of a romantic.
♡ Ask him who inspires him. Why? This will give you insight into what Mr. Libra finds attractive in other people.
♡ Ask him what injustices in the world upset him. How does he think it could be fixed? He's got definitive political and humanitarian opinions, and he'll appreciate a good discussion that focuses on these topics.
♡ Inquire about his family. He most likely has had family issues that made for much drama in his youth. Get the shocking

scoop early on, as this best gives you the barometer on how far he has come from it.

♡ Ask where he bought his outfit. Let loose with style and shopping talk. It'll seem vapid to anyone, but Libra.

♡ Bring up his pets. He loves animals and has a pet or fantasizes about getting one.

Music

Chances are high that your Libra plays a musical instrument, as they're all musicians at heart. If he isn't sonorously adept, his secret fantasy will involve being a virtuoso of some form or another. With that said, expect this will be reflective in his music tastes, as he'll tend to have vast and eclectic collection that dips into all genres—however, only worshipping the coolest of the cool. Libra prides himself on being up on the current trends and of course, knowing the hippest and most underground scenes. He's a total music aficionado in every sense of the word. Best to hide your embarrassing CDs before he comes over.

Mood Makers:

♡ Underground, hyper trendy, and/or hipster music. Show you're in the know, it'll turn him on.

♡ Classical. It's a safe romantic choice that can never go wrong.

♡ Foreign pop. It's highbrow if he doesn't know what they're singing about.

♡ Go-go music, lounge. Music that enhances the mood of cocktails can never be bad.

♡ Old jazz, blues, and soul. This appeals to Libra's inner musician.

♡ Samba. It's mellow enough to get him dancing, and close to you.

♡ Hall-of-fame music. Music that musicians respect are the cornerstones of his taste.

Gifts

Whatever you get him, it better look good and be of high quality, because giving him crap would be an insult too great for him to bear. Ideally, gifts he prefers will promote his idea of being a sophisticated and hip being, such as gifts that have a purpose for his creative pursuits or social climbing, or gifts that can be shared in some way. Also, presents with artistic merit will hit the spot—but no eyesores, thank you. Of course, being as gracious as they come, Libra will gladly accept any token of affection with a warm smile and have you believing it's divine. However, if you're not getting return calls to any of the many messages you've left, you shouldn't have to think hard to figure out why.

Boxed Treats:

♡ Well-designed pieces of home decor. He wants to surround himself in good aesthetics.

♡ Musical instruments or a mix CD. These presents can never get old with him.

♡ Clothes, cool labels please. They all have a fashion victim in them.

♡ Art. A photo, sculpture, music, painting, etc. Even better if it's your work. He extols artistic types.

♡ Tickets to a creative event—music preferably, but anything that's artsy will do.

♡ Supplies for his creative outlet. This treat shows your support.

♡ Throwing a social event in his honor. Memories with friends are priceless.

Touch Me

Libra perfected the art of seduction, making him the man who'd go limp in the face of low-class raunch or mid-tier bubbly. To please his senses, give him luxury love and be able to hold your own as a trophy piece looking for the same. To get him off, he'll need a well-balanced romantic partnership, starting with a cool image that translates into a lovely rapport. Optimum results will require you to be into smooth tag-team social climbing and possess a riveting amount of cultural curiosities that'll keep his mind hungry and his creative enthusiasm on the rise. You'll find that the sex will be his expression of that connection. The better you fulfill those duties, the better he'll perform for you.

Truth be told, he's not the horniest guy in the zodiac and he isn't driven by his libido. With him, it's the complete package of the relationship that'll drive his passion. The downfall is that it can get staid through time, as balance levels the lust off. This then leaves it to you to periodically shake it by opening sexual dialogues and unlocking the secrets. Creating a forum to share your fantasies and thinking new ones together will expand the boundaries of your lusty affairs and, in turn, his affection for you and your partnership. Sexual exploration is a trust matter with Libra, and the deeper your commitment gets, the easier and more enticed he'll be to dig deeper into the Pandora's box of sexual surprises.

Once you've entered into the great unknown, though, expect to be in charge of the adventure and encouragement quotient, while he complements the mix with his forte—which tends to come in the form of tenderness, romance, and the loving side to sex. Add an artsy overtone to the exchange for the ultimate way to arouse his senses, and seamlessly blend in his dirty desires with taste. Yes, think erotica, not porn. In no time, he'll slowly let go of his inhibitions and release the smutty slut inside of him that has been dying to break free, and when that occurs, you can bet that it'll be a most beautiful moment.

Ways to Heat Up Your Libra:

♡ Libras love to get their lower backs and ass stroked and cared for. Don't neglect this sensually delicate area as you travel on the road to forking over full body pleasure.

♡ Create a mix CD in which you both have to create sexual scenarios to match the songs.

♡ Use body paints or make genital sculptures of each other— integrate artistic expression and out you'll come with a sexy masterpiece.

♡ Have sex outdoors, preferably during sunrise or sunset.

♡ Dress up like an old-time movie star and surprise him some-where.

♡ Make art films or take photos during sex. Black and white of course.

♡ Roses and candles can never go wrong with him as long as you're the centerpiece with chilled champagne and lust in the air.

Role-playing

There's nothing Libra won't do in the name of art, even if it means putting on a harness. Yes, under his polite façade are plenty of nasty little fantasies. To ease them out of him, conceptualize your sex and set the stage for edgy scenes where he can break out of his repression. Whether his aspirations are of a soulful and artistic genius or a debonair playboy, his idols are the role-playing characters he'd like to inhabit. In playing them, it's like he's fucking you and them at the same time—a double bonus. Add any sort of creative tinge to the affair and you're thinking his kind of kink, like letting him film it. As soon as he calls, "Action," you'll discover he can be a total pig and a playful and disgusting one at that!

Cast of Characters:

♡ Supermodel and photographer. Anything involving beauty appeals to him.

♡ Rock star and stowaway groupie on a private jet. He's got a glam thing in him.

♡ Artist and muse. He is the sign of the artist.

♡ Jet-set spy and high-class hooker. This will speak to his suave side.

♡ Two principal dancers defecting from their troupe and finally reaching freedom. It's romantic and a little over the top.

♡ Unrequited lovers separated from war for years finally reuniting. It's a classic love story he'll love to indulge in.

♡ Two opposing attorneys getting their sexual tensions out after a heated day in court. Libras love to settle things out of court. They can make compromise hotter than you suspect.

Taking the Bait

When Libra feels connected, at its best, there's love, romance, and then more love and more romance. At worst, you'll gain a responsibility. Yes, the downside to this man is that his idea of commitment can mean becoming a co-dependent freak who needs you to sustain his lifeline. Just when you thought you met your Prince Charming who isn't afraid to talk about the future, you learn that the plans include being his parent and having to encourage him in every aspect of his life and to pay for it, too. This could leave you wondering where the Casanova went, as the dark side of a committed Libra is complacency. If this occurs, it'll usually be in a month— enough time to easily cut your losses, because this Libra isn't capable of loving you as much as he is of draining you. Of course, not all Libras are this way, but it happens more times than coincidence, so beware.

On the upside, if you surpassed the Libra curse and nabbed yourself a sweet one, then you'll know he's yours when he's consistently upping the ante to your bond and working on becoming a team with you. Expect things like your social calendar being filled into the next century as you busily keep up appearances while being part of his overbooked life. Yes, Libra is serious about being a couple, and jumping right in is the only way to see if the relationship will float. So, if the Siamese twin routine works for you and feeling like a married couple by the third date is cool, life will only get better. In time, you'll be his extension and he'll be attentive to you as he would himself, as he knows and lives to preserve the ideals of partnership. However, if this doesn't happen and he's not acting like your husband in a month, be leery of this Romeo's imminent departure, as acting as if he belongs to you is how he bonds with you.

UNAUTHORIZED: ASTRAL AUTOPSY

Recognizing Fear

Looking at Libra, no one would suspect behind that pretty little face is a neurotic freak, but surprise, surprise! As the sign of balance, Libra has spent his life trying to find his. To get to his current state, he most likely has gone through many minefields, either blindly walking into them or being shoved in. His past is typically somewhat dark and finding his center hasn't been easy. One of the ways he does anchor himself is with a partner—someone he can focus on instead of his demons or at least dilute his energies enough to quell his psychosis. Without another, it makes those voices in his head that much louder and scarier.

Main cause

Solitude.

Immunizing His Fears:

- ♡ Be as co-dependent as him and talk in "we" not "me" mode.
- ♡ Keep him in light social atmospheres; that's the type of environment he thrives best in.
- ♡ Always tell him he looks good before going out. He prides himself on this sense of style.
- ♡ Buy rounds for everyone. Generosity is a prime virtue he judges people on.
- ♡ Have a packed social calendar and always know where there's something happening—something cultural or hip. Antisocial or unfashionable people disturb him.

Infecting Him with Fear:

- ♡ Cancel plans last minute, when he's about to go somewhere new and no one else can escort him. He's not at ease flying solo.
- ♡ Expect him to make decisions quickly. Even things like choosing a movie with you will stress him out because he likes to weigh out options leisurely.
- ♡ Show up in a hideous outfit. He's horrified by bad taste, especially being seen with it.
- ♡ Stress you have to be somewhere at a certain time and force the punctuality issue—schedules make him feel claustrophobic.
- ♡ Have an emotional breakdown and pop anxiety pills (or placebos)—then freak out about running out of pills and how you can't book a second visit to your shrink during the week. He needs harmony and only wants to deal with his demons, not yours.

Recognizing Anger

Libra hates confrontations and will do anything to avoid them. He's the purveyor of justice and lives for harmony. After all, he's a lover, not a fighter. However, if there's no choice and he's forced to deal, he'll opt for solutions via logic and friendly compromises. Then, if his peaceful efforts go without acknowledgment or if they backfire, anger will be his last resort and a sign of his defeat. The worst thing about his rage is that it's sudden, making him snap and turning him into the Incredible Hulk. Expect all his pent-up anger to come rushing out, making it obvious why he has worked so hard to keep a lid on this ugly and consuming side to him. So, tread lightly!

Main cause
He can be a real sore loser.

Immunizing His Anger:

♡ Never jump to conclusions. Always listen to all sides of the story before losing your shit.

♡ Be loose and keep a carefree attitude toward everything.

♡ Share. All Libras are socialists and have no concept of sole ownership.

♡ If you need his help, suggest subtly, even if you're asking for help to avoid catastrophe. He won't respond to demands.

♡ In public, have manners suitable for royalty. Burping, talking loud, and things of that nature ruffle his feathers—don't do it!

Infecting Him with Anger:

♡ If you're going to one of his family or friend's celebrations (wedding, birthday, etc.), offer to buy the present. Then buy something ugly and put both your names on it. He'll be infuriated that you messed with his stylish reputation.

♡ Be cold to his pet. Libras tend to have an animal companion that they live and die for. Ignore them and he'll do the same to you.

♡ Refuse a communal atmosphere. Like, with a group dinner, insist on splitting the check exactly instead of evenly.

♡ Leave poor tips. He finds stinginess reprehensible.

♡ Borrow clothes and return them dirty. Not only is it rude, he'll be aghast that you were so disrespectful to his precious wardrobe.

Recognizing Sadness

Keeping a happy face is Libra's way, even when he's in pain. To him, sadness is a private matter and a shame. He's aware of how self-absorbed it is to indulge it, but he also understands it's a necessary evil—giving him a very pragmatic approach to ridding himself of it. To get out, he'll close himself off to dive deeper into his despair, until hitting rock bottom. Only when he's there will he get the momentum to spring back up and eventually settle back into contentment, therefore making sorrow a necessary route back to happy.

Main cause
There are no ups without downs.

Immunizing His Sadness:

♡ Love his friends as you love him. Remember to keep up that communal attitude.

♡ Do volunteer work. Just being with someone so kind and caring will make him act more so.

♡ Call him frequently and be his Siamese twin—co-dependence rocks with him.

♡ Always be ready to party. He'll typically respond well to being among people and music. He's a sponge for the energy of a festive social atmosphere.

♡ Keep his creative juice flowing; that's his life force.

Infecting Him with Sorrow:

♡ Want a private relationship with him and/or a social life that's separate from his.

♡ Drink soup with a straw or something just as déclassé. Bad manners upset him deeply and most likely will result in your dismissal, if you keep it up.

♡ Have no interest in his artistic abilities. He'll think you're just trying to avoid telling him that he has no talent.

♡ When you're out with him, cut out early from an event or place. Being left alone always makes him sad, but doing it abruptly will leave him no time to prepare and force him into solitude. He hates being alone.

♡ Have opposing political views from him. This is the one area he won't be able to compromise with this lover, and if you don't share his beliefs, he'll have to dump you.

Recognizing Trust

Generally, Libra believes people and the world are good. He thinks that by staying open to life and living fairly, he'll reap a pleasant one. However, he's no dummy and knows he also has to keep himself safe. Although he might invite the world into his life and be generous to a fault, he tends never to get too deeply involved with many people where a meaningful level of trust becomes an issue. He sees it unnecessary to give too much power, always maintaining a 50/50 boundary. His idea is that the bad seeds eventually weed themselves out, leaving him in the clear. Besides, as long as he's got his one good partner at his side, that'll be all he needs.

Main cause
How much do you need to trust someone to have a good time?

Immunizing His Trust:

♡ Invite him out everywhere. Have your life be an open house. Introduce him to all your friends right away and have them coo over him.

♡ Be into your looks. Image is important and he needs to know you're on his wavelength.

♡ Appreciate art. Libra considers anyone who doesn't a bore and those people can't be trusted.

♡ Always buy nice gifts for your loved ones, even if there's no occasion. He likes people who are kind all year long, not just when they have to be.

♡ Be on decent terms with your exes. How you dealt with past relationships reflects on your character.

Infecting His Sense of Trust:

♡ Turn into a total homebody. He'll think you're a creepy serial killer in the making.

♡ Love rules and adhering to them. He'll think you have no imagination. If you always do as you're told, he won't trust you know yourself.

♡ Be loud and brash. Socially clumsy people are untrustworthy because they won't know how to feel their environment and blend in gracefully. Libra has a zero tolerance on any ruckuses.

♡ Be emotional about making decisions that don't require emotions—like go out or order in. Your unpredictable emotional status will give him pause, as he only does smooth sailing.

♡ Be overly competitive. He won't trust anyone who causes pressure.

Recognizing Motivation

Libra does what he wants, when he wants. If it doesn't fall under the pursuit of leisure or helping restore peace in chaos or causing chaos in peace, he won't budge. Put demands on him and expect to be ignored, or worse, he'll do the opposite to spite you. Libra has his own time clock, does only what he feels, and no amount of pressure will change that. In fact, pressure shuts him off. Making suggestions without expectations is the only way you can hope he'll do as you wish because letting go of control is the first part in getting him to obey.

Main cause
Listening to his inner flow.

Immunizing His Motivation:

♡ Describe something as passé to stop him in his tracks. Being cool is his thing and he won't allow anything to tarnish his rep.

♡ Appeal to his sense of moral obligation. For example, if there's a restaurant he likes and you hate, then tell him they're violating their employees' rights.

♡ Bring him anywhere ugly and he'll shut down.

♡ If you hate something he's into, don't let him know. Tell him someone he obviously hates is into the same thing. It'll turn his stomach to share an interest with an unhip enemy. Like if he has an outfit you hate, say you saw it on so-and-so and it looked great on them.

♡ Enforce rigid rules or be demanding in a stern parental way. All Libras have had father issues and won't need to relieve them with you.

Infecting Him with Motivation:

♡ He's all for social causes. Anything for the less fortunate, he'll gladly help out.

♡ Tell him he's handsome and butter him up. Flattery is the remote control to his soul.

♡ Always hint at him when you want him to do something. The subtler, the more effective.

♡ If you make it sound exclusive, he'll show—whether it's a party or a dentist.

♡ The more people involved, the better chances he'll get involved. He likes to move with a group. Call it social or peer pressure, but it works.

DESTINATION: DUMPSVILLE

Celestial Voodoo on You

Libra hates to upset anyone, least of all himself. He'll do anything to avoid a confrontation and if that means ignoring you or disappearing, then so be it. It's not personal, that's just him. Once he feels an emotional disruption coming on, he'll withdraw himself until he finds a sense of calm. The time he does put into you, though, he'll act unsuspiciously. However, in his free time, he'll be out finding or courting another. His approach to a breakup is like trading in an old car; he'll use you up until he's picked out his next one.

He gets that ending a relationship is hard to do, and when one has gone its course, the best way to deal is run to another. With his new lover, Libra can look forward not backward. Besides, why bother thinking about a depressed and angry ex when there's a new and shiny lover to whom he can still be seen as perfect? Sure, it's diabolically selfish, but he's a relationship addict who is always out to find a bigger and better hit to satisfy his needs. Once one taste gets too tired, he has to find another fast, since going into withdrawal would be too hard to bear. It'll be at this moment, when you think back and see how he was so willing to commit, that it'll all make so much sense.

The upside is that when he's driving you to Dumpsville, it's obvious, if you want to see it. He'll gradually spend less time with you. Then, to make up for it, he'll shower you with spectacular gifts. He'll most likely buy you items that are more than he can afford; but realize this won't be your problem. Then, to assess the speed of his finale to the start of his new relationship, use the same timeline he used on you. His saving grace, though, is that he'll remain respectful of you and wait to sleep with that person until you're really out of the picture. He merely sets up a new nest when with you, but moves in when he's in the clear—as not cheating on you is what ultimately justifies his guilt.

. . . And Other Signs He Hates You

If Libra cares for you, he'll give you the benefit of the doubt. Being that he's as optimistic as they come, even if you abuse him, it'll take a while before it really registers with him because he's so programmed for peace. However, if you've struck out too many times and disrupted his psyche, expect him to snap back and to shut you out. Nobody messes with his balance, least of all your dumb ass, as he's had to endure too many challenges to achieve it. So, when he cuts you off, know it's his last option. Of course, being a gentleman through and through, he'll do it gracefully with one clean cut. If you try to resist, you'll learn coming onto unwelcome territory is futile. To keep up appearances, he'll always be kind, but will make it obvious it's out of sympathy. Libra has a gracious way about him, so know your humiliation is imminent. Also, being that he's a popular guy, he'll usually have a crowd with him that'll easily outnumber you, making you that much more invisible. With him, out of sight, out of mind, and voila, problem solved.

Beating Him to the Punch

No matter how many hints you give, Libra has a way of deflecting agony by playing dumb. He hears what he wants to hear and does whatever it takes to ignore anything obviously painful, even if it means procrastinating until death to accept an agonizing truth. This will hold doubly true when it comes to getting dumped unceremoniously. Typically, Libra will try to do whatever it takes to work it out rather than walk away. This could include your efforts or not, as he won't even see the difference.

To avoid any of that drama, forget even addressing any problems to Libra and just get too busy. Use work or family as your excuses so that you don't raise his suspicions. Just by the nature of spending less time with him, he'll naturally migrate to needing someone new to latch on to. Think of him like a magnet; his forces will eventually be drawn to a stronger and closer bond. Inevitably, he'll go away and move to a new lover. With this demise, it leaves you the option of making him feel guilty, too—which is just another bonus in sealing Libra's fate with this surefire passive-aggressive maneuver.

Ridding Yourself of Libra with Minimal Scarring:

- ♡ Be flirty with others in front of him. He's a natural flirt, but he's also a hypocrite.
- ♡ Look like hell and put little effort into your appearance when you get together and go out on the town.
- ♡ Want to stay at home and rot in front of the TV. Be negative, too, to add to the unalluring picture of the future he'll have with you.

♡ Be a buzz kill. Constantly enforce constraints on his wild behavior.

♡ Be stingy with cash and keep a tab on who spends what and on what.

♡ Suggest ugly decor for his place. It'll cut off any dreams he has of living with you.

♡ Communicate by nagging him.

Kick, Drop, and Kill

It's lonely after a romp with Libra, more so than any other breakup. With him, it's not just losing a boyfriend but also a scene. No matter how amicable the end, it's never a good idea to hang around after a breakup. Chances are he'll replace you shortly after (or has already). Or he'll eventually swing back to try to reignite the flames, starting a vicious cycle of failure. Either situation sucks. Save your ego and stay away.

While it's never easy after the good-byes, the nice thing about the Libra relationship postmortem is that he's not typically one of those lovers who makes you cringe when you do see him again—at least not in the span of a brief conversation. This makes it fabulous if you're strolling down the street sometime in your future with your new beau—which usually is a trifling situation, especially for the current love. Seeing your past up close and personal will make your new boyfriend wonder how he measures up. With Mr. Libra Cutie Pie, famous for his classic good looks and socially seductive savoir faire, he'll no doubt intimidate anyone who would have to walk in his footsteps. Sure, you might know the truth behind his supermodel gorgeousness, but it won't matter when it comes to making an impression on your new lover. It'll say a lot about you and your standards. It'll be in that moment, you'll finally bow down to the Libran way: Image is power, and hot damn, it feels good!

WANTED: SCORPIO

BORN OCTOBER 23—NOVEMBER 21

Master manipulator with a starry gaze that can transfix objects directly to its genitals. When provoked, its poison sting will cause permanent damage.

BARE BASICS

How to Spot Him

You can feel a heat radiating to you from across the room. You look up, scan, and magnetically lock eyes with him. He stands still, inconspicuously emanating his presence amid some raucous scene and shooting forth a power of sex appeal that reaches into your deepest curiosities. His alluring stance commands an intensity that makes him irresistible, and you come hither. You slowly move toward him; a heat spills into your panties and moisture marks your anticipation. Unbeknown to you, this has been your first sting of Scorpio.

Ahh, Scorpio, the sign of mystery, the silent Casanova, the unrelenting enigma that swings between love god and cocky asshole, but always sexy. He never fails to impress in life, love, and especially in girth and length. Typically endowed with a pleasantly plump member that lures him in and out of treachery with excruciating desire, his salvation is that he's bestowed with an intensity that can be fiercely healing on one hand, manipulative, and psychotic on another. It's all about how he chooses to balance himself, which usually is a lifetime struggle.

With seemingly no middle ground to his psyche, Scorpio plays the perfect big ole misunderstood bitch. He resists showing the man behind the curtain, preferring you to see him as a magical wizard who can make anything happen. Of course, no one can pull that off without a serial killer mentality—and for many Scorpios, that's a birthright. Masked behind a secret agent façade, he's frequently seen as cold, selfish, evil, or a combo of all three. With power and pride always on the line, a Scorpio won't reveal more than necessary. His heart is an exclusive club and not even a blow job to the bouncer will get you past his emotional velvet ropes (but he'll appreciate the attempts nonetheless). It's VIP guest list all the way.

In wielding this strong and musky animal magnetism, he'll approach his mating grounds quietly. Reclusive by nature, Scorpio doesn't generally like large and unfamiliar situations. Usually he'll slink in, sum up the scene, find his place, and look for something to hold on to before letting go. Whether it's a person or his ninth cocktail, comfort kicks in only when he has a security blanket. Then, after gaining familiarity, he'll turn to territorializing his ego all over the area, acting out in all sorts of ways that can be caring or conniving.

If you're the soul that's courageous or insane enough to take on this dashing devil, realize Scorpio is an all or nothing kind of guy. His quest is to find that one-in-a-trillion lover to cash out his jackpot of infinite and transcendental love, and to have even one roll with him means high stakes, as he dwells in a world of extremes. With a history typically marked with many casualties, understand it's no easy task attempting to taste the passion from which legends are made. However, with odds as sexy as these, who could resist? Certainly no one with any backbone.

Key Features:

♡ Usually adorned in dark colors, a dramatic look or some kind of costume/uniform

♡ A deep, penetrating stare
♡ A mysterious aura
♡ Sex appeal seemingly oozing from every pore
♡ A loner vibe
♡ A dirty mouth that'll spew many sexual innuendos
♡ A secretive way of communicating

Seducing Him into Your Boudoir

Bagging a Scorpio is a hit-or-miss game. He's a first-instinct kind of guy and assigns his prey's sexual fate immediately, but being the man he is, he'll still flirt with any hag regardless of intention. Sexual attention is sexual attention and anyone is welcome to worship the Adonis known as Scorpio. If you think you have what he wants, call him on one of his many sexual innuendos. Most likely armed with a potty mouth, he'll make several sexual suggestions in conversation—no matter what the topic of discussion. Prove you've got the chutzpah to take him on by whipping back a dose of sexual banter filled with ten times more smut. If he's interested, this will give him a hard-on like you wouldn't believe.

If your response falls on deaf ears, go find someone else to appreciate your sexy wit ASAP. Understand that going closer to a fire that doesn't want to ignite your passions may cause an invitation for you to dance with a flame, which will leave you charred rather than cherished. Scorpios love power, and if he finds a way to dominate you through desire, he'll find this just as tasty as fucking—but the only person getting off is him. So use caution: Scorpios screw in many ways, so be responsible for your actions.

Once nabbed, though, match his enthusiasm and you'll get the stuff of XXX cinema. He likes to talk dirty, so follow his lead and do the same. Let your fantasies and secrets spill out; they are his aphrodisiac. Scorpio understands the submission of your sexual thoughts breed trust, making him feel as if he has the biggest balls on the block. So, play to win with this bad boy by walking the walk, talking the talk, and being fearlessly sexual.

Loving Him in the Boudoir

Where there's sex, there's Scorpio. However, despite his reputation as a 24-7 horn dog that's all about his cock, know that he has a propensity to be a loudmouth bottom. Yes, the secret's out: Although Scorpios are preoccupied with sex, it isn't always a physical desire as much as it's a cerebral one for control. He knows desire makes the world go round, and the most potent and primal desire is sexual. Therefore, sex is power. The dumber Scorpios take this literally and justify it by thinking with their dicks. The smarter ones use this belief both literally and metaphorically to succeed in all they do. However, both strive for excellence, determined to be legendary lovers to all of their conquests—fucking to impress and getting off on immortalizing themselves in your genital memory.

So, if you're feeling horny, dive right in. The sex is never bad, as his reputation is on the line each and every time. Expect the utmost intensity, passion, decadence, and drama. Scorpio's approach to sex is like an opening night of a theatrical debut, with you as his critic giving him a review that can make or break him. With the pressure on (at least in his mind), he'll bring in everything he's got to give a performance worthy of front-page headlines. This all goes back to his need for absolute acceptance, which is his curse. However, how it works out in the sack is just lovely for you, as nothing is ever off limits and victory is always a must. With ambitions like his, everyone comes a winner.

Plus, with such a big cock, who could resist? Scorpio gives sex that lingers, leaving an imprint you won't forget (just allow yourself some time to snap back into place, literally) . . . Yes, even if he isn't tops with technique, he makes up for it with his wonderfully sized cock and fetish for sex and power. He rarely leaves any unsatisfied customers.

MAKING HIM COME TO THE PALM OF YOUR HAND

Eye Candy

Scorpios get hard on drama and power. Think a toned-down Alexis Carrington of *Dynasty* and you've got the prototype for Scorpio's desires. To pull off this look of survivor bitch, think black and minimal, fitted with clean lines and sexy cuts—and throw in as much je ne sais quoi as you can. Scorpio wants his lover to ooze with sex appeal, making him look as if he's a man of power. Do your part by showing some skin, carrying your sexuality confidently and charming coolly and cruelly.

Stylin' Seduction:

♡ Black and red. Black because it exudes power, mystery, and the unknown. Red because it's the color of victory, passion and blood. All things that Scorpio adores.

♡ Solid colors. Scorpios are low key and don't like to stand out with loud prints.

♡ Stylish vintage outfits. It can never go wrong with him. Scorpios love retro styles.

♡ Look like a stylishly smart asset as he yearns to be half of a power couple. If he's a businessman, go all out with labels and power suits. If he's an artist, wear the trendiest and most underground designers. If he's a non-profiteer, think organic fiber panties.

♡ Expensive labels. He won't readily admit it, but it turns him on. Money is power.

♡ Hair. He loves a vixen with great bed head.

♡ He's all about costumes, so play up your style with themes— such as military, peasant, or sexy librarian.

Tasty Treats

Food

Scorpio is particular. He won't put just anything in his mouth. As far as food, he can be quite a bore, tending to stick to the tried and true—as in food he grew up with or anything fairly uncomplicated on the palette. If he happens to get curious, he'll try to get you to order that new dish, as the commitment is just too much for him. Sure, it's shockingly uninspiring, but he's loyal in every way, even down to his last taste bud.

Erotic Eats:

♡ Traditional dining halls that have a lodge feel to them. Scorpios love that old-world feeling.

♡ A roadside greasy spoon with lots of character/characters. Anything with a B-movie feel, he'll love.

♡ Waterfront seafood joints. He loves seafood and he loves water views; put them together and it spells fun. Plus, he's a water sign.

♡ A bedroom picnic with lots of finger foods. It's all his favorite things to eat in one place.

♡ Fondue (in the nude for extra fun!). It's sexy and romantic in that '70s swinger kind of way.

♡ Any cozy home-cooking restaurant. He digs lowbrow ambiances and no-nonsense food.

♡ A trendy and underground restaurant with a waiting list you have the power to pass. Impress him with your ability to pull strings.

Movies

Hot and heady porn is a way to jolt Scorpio's attention. Put it on, and within minutes of the libidinous celluloid rolling, you'll have an engorged Scorpio in front of the boob tube. However, if you want to save the XXX adventure for a later date, keep it light with Mr. Intensity. Comedy is good. Black comedy is even better. Avoid dramas in the "get to know you" phase; they can cause an emotional tension that'll make him (and you) uncomfortable. Best choices would be horror or suspense. He loves to show off his ability to handle gore and dementia, and it'll give him lots to talk about. After, he'll ramble on and on about how he would have perfected the murders, been a better psycho, or outsmarted evil.

Cinematic Foreplay:

♡ Horror flicks. Preferably stick to films featuring satanic themes and/or supernatural elements and/or serial killers. He'll relate to these as if there were bios.

♡ Suspense. He's the sign of mystery!

♡ Melodrama. Anything intense, he's all over it.

♡ Black comedy. Scorpio's attitude: Laughing at someone is better than laughing with them.

♡ Erotica. It's close to porn.

♡ Violent movies. The bloodier, the better.

♡ Disaster flicks. Don't be surprised if he laughs at the most gruesome scenes; he's disturbed like that.

Dating Ideas

To woo a Scorpio, plan self-revealing activities. Scorpio shows himself surreptitiously and likes to uncover info the same way. Charm the boots off him at locales that express creativity and depth. Bring him somewhere meaningful to you. If you expose part of your history, Scorpio will appreciate the gesture and may even return one to you. However, always avoid any large group activity in uncharted territory.

There's nothing worse for Scorpio than the possibility of coming off as a fool. Pride is his co-pilot and he hates looking like a novice. Plus, giving exclusive attention is crucial to putting Scorpio at ease. He's all about being focused on you and you being focused on him. Besides, why would anyone resist being the star under this sex god's seductive stare?

Playful Planning:

- ♡ A haunted house, picnic at a cemetery, or any spooky-themed activities. Anything dealing with the occult fascinates him.
- ♡ Your favorite dive bar. Be warned though, most Scorpios are bad drunks.
- ♡ A water park or any water-themed locale. Being around water brings out his romantic side.
- ♡ Sex club or sex-themed activity. Anything involving sex is an endless fascination with him.
- ♡ A visit to a psychic or an astrologer. It'll be a good way to pry info out of him without asking.
- ♡ A drive-in movie theater. It offers privacy with entertainment.
- ♡ Cave exploration or any underground activity—literally and metaphorically. He loves dark and musky places.

Sound Seduction

Conversation

Scorpio wants to get deep inside people in more ways than sexual. Superficial banter makes him ill, and he appreciates anyone who can cut to the chase and share who they really are. Go ahead: Dive in with profoundly personal questions. Topics that make him purr include your sexual history, philosophies, and survivor stories. There's nothing more erotic to him than knowing you've been to hell and back—a journey he knows all too well.

Icebreakers:

- ♡ Ask when he lost his virginity. He'll love reminiscing about this major turning point.
- ♡ Find out the kinkiest place he's done it and learn how anal he is or isn't.
- ♡ Discuss his sexual fantasies, ones he's lived out and ones he has yet to—and be prepared to listen all night.
- ♡ Find out what he wants his funeral to be like. Scorpio rules death and is obsessed with it, by way of fear or fascination.
- ♡ Ask about his traumatic experiences. This will reveal his depth level.
- ♡ Ask him if he would rather die drowning or burning. Any "would you rather" questions work, as you can uncover personal facts playfully. Morbid ones are his favorites.
- ♡ Ask him about his experiences with drugs. This will tend to rattle the skeletons in his closet into popping open that door.

Music

Drama, drama, drama! Music that's dark, decadent, and on the brink of destruction or ecstasy puts Scorpio in the mood. Songs with openly sexual themes, put them on! Any form of sexual suggestion will hypnotically put him right where you need him. Just turn it up, and he'll come right to the palm of your hand.

Mood Makers:

- ♡ Melancholy and dramatic music. The more morbid, the better.
- ♡ Requiems, bagpipes, Dixieland. Anything you might hear at a funeral, put it on. This is the sign of death.
- ♡ Dance music. Anything that can get your body moving will excite him.
- ♡ Music of his youth, whatever time that was and whatever was popular. Scorpios love nostalgia.

♡ Jazz vocalists. Only those that are long dead, though, and sing about what drove them to their demise. Music revealing that artist's self-destructive passions will turn him on.

♡ Rumba, samba, bossa nova or anything sultry sounding. It'll bring out his sex kitten.

♡ Soundtracks. Dramatic foreign ones tend to be the best suited for his passionate tastes.

Gifts

Scorpio considers gifts a subliminal message on how you perceive him, so choose wisely. Invest time to think about what you want to express, and recall all the details Scorpio has filled you in on. If you step back, you'll most likely see that he has been hinting what he wants all the while. It's all about subtlety with this one, so stay alert, as his expectations are always high. Yes, your ability to piece together the small details will say everything to Scorpio—and know there's a heavy price to be paid if you don't send the message he wants to hear.

Boxed Treats:

♡ A nude photo of you. Who could resist this one?!

♡ Detective paraphernalia. He loves mystery, and all Scorpios are snoops by nature.

♡ Paranormal books/tools. Scorpios rule the occult.

♡ Sex toys. Hello, figure this one out yourself.

♡ Costumes for role-playing. It's something for you and him.

♡ A diary. It makes a great outlet for his disturbing thoughts.

♡ Anything that's monogrammed or customized. He's a territorial creature.

Touch Me

Sex is everything for Scorpio. He's passionate and wants to get lost in the sex, be reborn in it, and transform you while he's at it. He wants it with all the intensity of the universe wrapped up in one orgasmic bundle of fun. So, don't hold back with him. Throw in all your enthusiasm and liberate your libido, because once you dive into the sack with Scorpio, it's judgment day. Sex is no joke for Scorpio because it is the testing ground for whether you stay or go.

Make sex as adventurous as possible and bend the rules. Go ahead, make it dirty—he'll want you more. Live to shock. The more daring the ideas, the more your chemistry will meld into an unforgettable bumping of the uglies. Feel free to break out the porn, sex toys, duct tape, or whatever else you have to titillate. Going to the extremes is what turns him on, and a lover with a sexually courageous attitude is his idea of a good time. Whatever taboos you have, spill them out and let him break them. If he can play your sexy super-hero, liberating you from repression, this will get him off even more. So, don't be shy! Scorpio usually has had lots of sex; by making your talents and abilities stand out, it'll be just the spice he'll want to taste.

As for the body part that he'll want you to give all the attention to, think dick (like you didn't know already?!). Then, if he's well behaved, add ass to the game. While foreplay is great, instant insertion is way hotter. If the sex is hot, the foreplay can follow. After all, he has to know what he's getting into and what to be inspired for, so he can keep rising to that occasion.

However, if all this sounds foreign to the Scorpio you snagged, think twice before going any further. Safety tip #1: avoid any Scorpios who are no longer virgins and still uptight about sex. Unfortunately, there are a few out there. As the sign of sex and extremes, Scorpios fall to either side of the sexual liberation fence. If your Scorpio falls to the lame side, run while you can. A non-sexually liber-ated Scorpio is the fifth horseman of the Apocalypse and you need to back away from the danger ASAP, as you don't need his issues blowing up all over you.

Ways to Heat Up Your Scorpio:

- ♡ Scorpio's erogenous zone is his genitals, but don't heat it up too fast. Tease him with a light ball massage, or dry hump-ing. It'll make him too hot to handle!
- ♡ He loves his secrets, so make a play for him at a large get-together and discreetly find a spot to do it in.
- ♡ He's a water sign, do him near a body of water. It'll make him super-hot.
- ♡ Send him handcuffs in the mail with an invitation of the time and place he can use them.
- ♡ Make your own porn together.
- ♡ Do him in a bar bathroom at least once in your relationship.
- ♡ Get him a cock ring with your name monogrammed on it. He'll love that you think of him as a sexual possession.

Role-playing

Scorpio is a natural role-player, as he already hides behind masks in someway or another. For sex though, he's upfront about wanting a role-playing partner in crime. His preferred theme: power. He knows domination and submission is the way of the world, so why hide it in the bedroom? Take the S & M theme beyond the traditional leather and whips to create scenes where power intermingles with imagination. Remember, you're dealing with the slut of the zodiac: Keep his interests erect by flexing your creativity muscle forcefully. He's all about the psychological special effects of sexual theater— so make it as original as you can and be the director with the award-winning scenes.

Cast of Characters:

- ♡ Mortician and corpse. Other people's idea of gruesome is Scorpio's aphrodisiac.
- ♡ Assassin and spy. He loves secrets.
- ♡ Royal leader and peasant. Power always makes him hot.
- ♡ Vampire and mortal. Again, the variation on the death theme will appeal to Scorpio.
- ♡ Prostitute and customer. Sleazy sexual themes appeal to him.
- ♡ Drug dealer and addict. Desperation turns him on.
- ♡ Beauty pageant contestant and wayward judge. Another variation on the power theme that can't ever go wrong with him.

Taking the Bait

Scorpio only clicks with someone who has the precise combo of charm, patience, and power to unlock his abandon. If you've got what it takes, this once seemingly distant creature will open up petal-by-petal right in front of you. He'll start by sharing the skeletons in his closet one by one. Then, he'll follow it with a flood of intensity that'll fill you with passionate devotion and a feeling of fated happiness. He doesn't readily share his emotions, so when he does, know he means it. Giving a compliment might be easy for some, but Scorpio sees it as a badge of honor that must be earned.

In the sack, he'll aim to please you for you and not his ego. He'll give you sex that'll make your ass sweaty in the middle of winter on top of an ice block in Antarctica. Yes, he'll love you completely, intensely, and vigorously. He won't settle for anything less than a cosmic connection and complete possession. When he submits, his love is impossible to contain. He'll want to give you the world and will do anything for you. Hell, he might even apologize when he knows he's wrong. Of course, he'll always have his private issues and an irrational belief that allows him to act as if he's a universal dictator who commands the last word on everything. Yet, despite all his Queenie behavior, the love he can dish out is gratifying, and Scorpio will let you know how much you are needed/wanted back with a positivity that'll pulsate in and out of your loins and right into your soul.

With all that said, as Scorpio's #1, you better take that duty seriously because Scorpio hates to be proven wrong. In a crisis, you'll be the first one he'll call—and you had better have some answers and comfort no matter what time he needs you. Plus, to indulge his suspicious mind, he'll give crisis drills every so often to assure himself of your capabilities and his judgment. That's right: Even in love, manipulation will still seep into the picture. There's a fine line between good and evil for Scorpio, and oftentimes he won't know how to stop himself from stepping over that line. It's this fact that makes them the most hated/misunderstood sign of the zodiac.

The final frontier in conquering Mount Scorpio is when he introduces you to everyone he knows. His presentation of you validates his commitment. Sharing you makes a statement to others, revealing something about him that means everything to him. Yes, once you're no longer Scorpio's secret, know you're loved.

UNAUTHORIZED: ASTRAL AUTOPSY

Recognizing Fear

Fear is the ultimate four-letter word to Scorpio, an emotional apocalypse and a complete loss of control. He usually finds himself in this disconcerting situation when his passions have run amok and his instincts have failed. Generally not a spontaneous type and calculating everything to the last, when things go off route Scorpio tends to go haywire and then begins to question his judgment completely.

At this uncertain crossroad, he'll feel uncomfortably open to ridicule and see fight or flight as his only options. What he chooses will be a gauge of his real character as he'll either whip out his inner reserves of strength or his inner ruthless asshole. Who pops out could be anyone's guess.

Main cause
Being unable to predict the future with 100 percent accuracy.

Immunizing His Fears:

♡ Never call him out when he hits a rut; Scorpio has a poker-face do-it-alone approach. You have to be invited to partake in his fears; otherwise he'll think you don't think he's capable.

♡ Scorpio thinks of himself as perfect. Promote the madness by sacrificing a scapegoat and throwing the blame on someone else. It'll always bring him back onto solid ground.

♡ Fear is often his excuse for self-destructive behavior. As represented by the Phoenix, sometimes he must hit rock bottom to rise to the top. Throw him an extravagant denial party to bounce him back.

♡ Break out the Ouija. As the sign ruling the occult, he's not scared to go to the beyond to get answers.

♡ Never forget he's the sign of sex. His balls grow each time he plays his part as Cock Master of the Universe: invincible to the last drop. Blindside him with some good lovin' to jiggle his brain back into place.

Infecting Him with Fear:

♡ When he asks for information or advice, give it to him. Then, a few hours or days after, change your mind. This undermines his ability to differentiate right from wrong and strategize his defenses, leaving him vulnerable.

♡ Ask to borrow something of his. He'll hate saying no, but he's too territorial to easily say yes. He'll probably offer to buy you one rather than lend his out.

♡ Invade his space. He'll be worried you'll uncover one of his skeletons. Even if you aren't a snooping type, he'll fear you'll turn into one. He's all about possibilities—paranoid possibilities—so fuck with his mind.

♡ Cite his physical quirks as possible symptoms for rare, possibly fatal, but always chronic diseases that you "read about." Scorpios are hypochondriacs. If he's one of those neat-freak Scorpios, take away his antibacterial wipes and point out germs for kicks.

♡ Have a friend of yours he never met say, "Oh, I know all about you" with a smirk on their face. Scorpio's immediate response will be to demand to know what that person has heard. Have this individual then withhold the info and drive Scorpio nuts with anxiety.

Recognizing Anger

Just like an earthquake, it takes a lot of time and pressure before Scorpio erupts. As a sideways communicator, pinpointing his anger requires listening with the sensitivity of a seismograph. While brewing his anger, he'll keep a placid exterior. He stays silent because he knows everyone has the right to live the way they want, despite his feelings. However, he thinks people are aware of their own bad behavior and will correct it through his telepathic anger. Failing to see that people can't read his mind, Scorpio explodes and there's no telling to what extreme of anger he'll go. Attacks are usually sudden and always damaging.

Main cause
Feeling as if he's been let down or disregarded.

Immunizing His Anger:

- ♡ Confront Scorpio head-on to circumvent the anger. Diplomacy will work with him and catch him off guard.
- ♡ Be a bit possessive and jealous. He'll love your passion.
- ♡ If you know you're in the wrong, make emotional excuses for your behavior and bare your soul. He'll be too touched by your vulnerability to even think about getting upset.
- ♡ Always keep him informed. Absolve yourself of his suspicious nature that can incite his anger.
- ♡ Scorpios need overwhelming attention periodically and use anger as a cry for attention, so drop everything at a moment's notice and fulfill this desire. It should take only a few hours and 90 percent of your life force, as he'll begin to feel vulnerable soon enough and slink off toward a loner mentality.

Infecting His Anger:

- ♡ Copycat his behavior or ideas, but pass them off as yours. He hates being robbed of anything he feels is his and anyone who can't get their own ideas.
- ♡ Never let him control the music in the car or have any say over the little things.
- ♡ Tell someone he hates that he likes them—lies like these enrage him beyond repair.
- ♡ Make him wait. While he may waste your time, he expects you to respect his. For him, waiting is comprised of painful seconds that jab at his abandonment issues. He'll despise you for making him go there.
- ♡ Scorpio likes his things where they are, so shift his knickknacks around, remove things, place them elsewhere and watch him go insane!

Recognizing Sadness

As the sign of extremes, Scorpio does nothing half-assed, including bouncing around the emotional spectrum at full throttle. However, being that he doesn't readily express these vast emotions, yet expects everyone to know what he's feeling, it can cause his depression to heighten to a place where he'll have convinced himself that he's really desperate and pathetic—and it won't matter how popular he is the rest of the time, as every moment is a life-and-death matter unto itself. So, unless he's showered with love 24-7 without question, forget it, it's inevitable that he'll have to spend some nights crying himself to sleep.

Main cause
Inability to be everyone's #1 priority.

Immunizing His Sadness:

♡ Talk about your problems with him first and let him know that. He loves feeling needed.

♡ Be obsessed with him and love him as if he were your cult leader.

♡ Gossip. Giving him the exclusive goods on people more messed up than him always picks him up.

♡ Bring him somewhere where he's better than a majority of the people—as in better looking, more successful, smarter. A false boost to his ego always works well with him.

♡ Have an evil sense of humor; that'll keep him in good spirits.

Infecting Him with Sorrow:

♡ Get his pet to like you more than him. If he has a pet, he'll love it more than he'll ever love you—get him jealous and he'll go manic for sure.

♡ Talk about plans and don't invite him. Don't even apologize for this behavior. While most other people would ask why they have been excluded, Scorpio will respect that it's your choice and sulk in silence—letting the pain settle deep into his dark and bottomless soul.

♡ When going away, put him in a B&B instead of booking a hotel. Upset him by robbing the role of anonymous stranger from him—which is how be prefers to be on vacation.

♡ Before giving him a gift, make a big deal over it. Meanwhile, buy a gift that isn't him at all. It'll upset him to think you really don't understand him.

♡ Ask everyone but him for advice, and have him overhear this fact. If you disregard his opinion once, he'll think you never cared.

Recognizing Trust

Trust is what makes Scorpio's world go round. Giving it out is based on his intuition, and when he's feeling it his guard comes down, allowing him to safely be himself and melt into you. Usually this utterly magical and destined connection will manifest itself in the sack—the one place he feels he can express himself openly. Of course, as soon as he zips up his pants, the trust may end. Therefore, use your better judgment when dealing with this sign that's symbolized by an ugly and poisonous animal.

Main cause
Really seeing the individual or situation in question and still liking what results.

Immunizing Him with Trust:

♡ Be natural. Scorpio is not for amateurs. He's born with an infallible sixth sense and will rip to shreds anyone who tries to pose their way into his heart.

♡ Remember the details he has shared with you. He trusts anyone who's a good listener, like him, as it shows your character.

♡ Acknowledge his quirks. By showing you understand and care for him, you earn his trust.

♡ Have a policy of honesty over politeness; otherwise he'll see you as weak for wanting to be nice at any cost.

♡ Have more power than Scorpio. He may not really trust you, but he'll have to—as he's so mesmerized by power, he'll do anything to be around it.

Infecting His Sense of Trust:

♡ Psych him out. It doesn't take a brain surgeon to get Scorpio suspicious; he came out of the womb this way. Get caught in a white lie once and he will never forget it.

♡ Follow the rules. This is the mark of a cog-mentality and a suck-up, very bad in Scorpio's eyes. Trusting you means trusting your judgment.

♡ Be late. Even if he isn't on time himself, he'll expect you to be. If you don't respect his time, he won't believe you really appreciate him. With that, he won't ever be able to trust you completely.

♡ Be prudish and keep him suspicious. If you aren't open about sex in some way, shape, or form, Scorpio will probably not even like you, let alone trust you.

♡ Be overly subservient to him. Anyone he feels has no backbone is a parasite and deemed untrustworthy in every sense of the word—even if he was the one who set the trap.

Recognizing Motivation

Inspiration needs to come from a higher power before Scorpio takes action. He's the type who thinks everything he does is part of some grand scheme—so motivation needs to go down deep, way past superficial reasons. However, once focused, this man is indomitable and can make the impossible happen.

Main cause

Vision—any divine inspiration. Everything is a life-and-death matter, even getting off his ass.

Immunizing His Motivation:

- ♡ He looks for signs, so make up stuff and tell him it's a prediction. It's amazing how gullible he is to the letters E.S.P.
- ♡ Any activity that could be rated PG 13 is not for him.
- ♡ If it involves anyone he hates, count him out. He'd rather eat dirt than absorb bad energy voluntarily.
- ♡ Put him under a spotlight and give him an audience. It'll make him avoid the situation like a disease.
- ♡ Give him an ultimatum; there's nothing more disturbing to him. Then, watch him self-destruct to spite you. Let him have the battle, while you take the war.

Infecting Him with Motivation:

- ♡ Never directly demand, plant ideas. Scorpio doesn't like taking orders from anyone.
- ♡ Brag about him. Nothing moves him like living up to the idol you made him out to be.
- ♡ Anything underground, dangerous, exclusive, or a secret, he'll want a piece of without question.

♡ An activity that can test his endurance, sign him up. He loves proving his persistence.

♡ Tell him something is sexy and he's in

DESTINATION: DUMPSVILLE

Celestial Voodoo on You

Scorpio is a control freak. If you can't co-exist with his rules in a way he can appreciate, expect to be dumped. If you were merely a nuisance to him, he'll dispose of you quickly. If you affected him, he'll torture you slowly and steadily before giving in. The deeper he feels pained, the longer the misery he'll impose by way of psychological warfare. However, he'll keep it subtle enough to leave you wondering if you're just being paranoid. Trust your instincts always. His method is always to opt for the mind-fuck if he can.

After all, mental torture is Scorpio's hobby and passive-aggressive behavior is his vehicle. Instead of dumping you swiftly and responsibly, he prefers to fumble back and forth for long periods—weighing out options as if he were God. Meanwhile, he'll treat you like an emotional guinea pig, testing his abilities to read you like a book and subtly jabbing your soft spots when he feels like it. He'll zoom in on all your vulnerabilities and make hurtful "observations." If he really despises you, he'll pride himself on tearing you down in fifteen syllables or less when he can. He'll sniff out your issues, pry them out of your head, wrap them into a topsy turban, and squeeze your ego dry. His motto in war: "It's not only that I win, but that others lose."

The worst part about Scorpio is his obsession with power means loving revenge with the same eagerness. In causing any agitation with him, even the anguish of thinking he has to dump you, he'll feel the need to avenge justice for his duress. Plus, if Scorpio feels he has a part of you that he can control, his addiction to that power may be overwhelming and can make things even trickier. So, at the end, expect him to be desperate in his actions. He understands that a master without a servant is no one, and handing over his title is never simple. In fact, it can be extremely disturbing to go there with Scorpio, as his dementia and unrelenting ways are unpredictable. At the core, he'll plow down anyone with an obnoxious lack of emotion until he has won without a shadow of a doubt or until someone dies. If it's the former, the finale is when Scorpio attempts to regain his composure, which will mean covering his tracks. Of course, the first place he'll throw the dirt is over his memories of you.

. . . And Other Signs He Hates You

Scorpios keep it on the down low—except when they hate you. He has no problem expressing his negative emotions. In fact, that fucker may even be flamboyant about it. The more he hates you, the more attention you'll get. If he hates you mildly, he'll simply erase you from his renowned memory. The fact is that if he uses this method, he actually held no respect for you. To hate you, he needs 100 percent of his energy to be consumed by disturbed thoughts of you. Sure, it's insulting to be quickly forgotten, but be glad you get off this easy.

If he does despise you and curses the day you were born, he'll spend night and day rallying others to hate you, even people who may not know you. For those he finds absolutely despicable, Scorpio will create a custom-tailored program of vile thoughts, images, and secrets (and even rumors with the truly unscrupulous Scorpios) to create a behind-the-scenes mass hysteria against you. Watch out, as he sabotages quietly. His main goal: Make the object of his repulsion completely unfuckable. For him, "castration" is the worst form of torture, and when on his shit list, he'll castrate you to anyone who could possibly care.

Beating Him to the Punch

Scorpio teeters on a very delicate balance of sanity, which means he's easy to destroy for those not faint of heart. The problem, though, he transforms just as quickly and then lives to retaliate—even if it means spending every penny and the rest of his life torturing the shit out of you. Revenge is an ability Scorpios were born to perfect—so be careful. If possible, make the break quick and clean from this mind trap, because an unorganized plan of retreat will result in you becoming another statistic in Scorpio's quest for true love.

If you need to see him suffer, there's one simple solution: Disregard his existence. You know that saying, "Living the good life is the best revenge." Well, that was meant to pierce the heart of a Scorpio. He wants to see his enemies in pain. If you seem to recover from his passion with ease, he'll think he had no effect on you—making him feel invisible and powerless, which strikes at his biggest fear: being forgotten. So, understand if you really want to get him back, as in gutting his soul, it'll take time. Consider that karmic "bumping into each other moment" post-breakup to be your most potent payback time. Be kind and even caring, but make it apparent that you've moved on. Condescension delivered off-handedly is a dagger right to the heart, a bullet to the back, impotence. Even if you didn't date him long, this will still irritate the hell out of him. It's easy and like playing possum: Lie there and relax as you go in for match point against this master of deception.

Ridding Yourself of Scorpio with Minimal Scarring:

♡ Act unenthused in bed or fall asleep right before any action is to begin. He'll take this personally and get rid of you to ease his humiliation.

♡ Snoop through Scorpio's things and get caught. You'll be excused faster than you can spell "psycho."

♡ Be nice to his enemies. A Scorpio finds that kind of behavior reprehensible.

♡ Forget his birthday or any of his special events. He'll be too sensitive to deal.

♡ Impose rules on him and be serious about it. Nobody tells Scorpio what to do.

♡ Be caught checking out other men you know he would be intimidated by. Get him at his ego.

♡ Stand him up in public or publicly humiliate him in some way. He gives no second chances once this happens.

Kick, Drop, and Kill

It's easy to know when you've reached the end with Scorpio. He'll shoot his deadly stare so psychically deep into you, that you get his message and know to watch your back. As the most unrelenting member of the zodiac, fully eradicating a Scorpio can take a long time—sometimes even longer than your entire relationship. Why? His emotions run deep and he's unable to rest until he feels he's gotten his just deserts (aka the psychological slitting of your throat as his ego trophy). However, know that how he goes about rectifying his "peace" will be random and unpredictable. It may be relatively innocuous or it may be years later, after he's created some master sabotage, that he'll resurface to cause havoc. Yes, Scorpio can really be this demented.

Whatever the case: Avoid contact. If you don't, Scorpio will keep pouring salt over your wounds until you're turned inside out and bled of any reason. Realize, Scorpio doesn't have any sense of genuine diplomacy, especially when he can't even control the venom oozing from the sides of his mouth as he blabbers about how sincere he really may or may not be. Plus, the worst part is you can't predict the degree of passion Scorpio will put into avenging his hurt, making him a loose cannon who is as enigmatic as he is deadly. So, the moral of this tale: Don't waste your time on this one unless you've got a strong constitution and you're willing to go to hell and back, as that's the only way Scorpio travels.

WANTED: SAGITTARIUS

BORN: NOVEMBER 22—DECEMBER 21

Spastic pop-eyed idealistic wild child on a constant hunt for a catharsis. Speaks as if he's on a pulpit, with or without an audience. Always open to suggestions, but never about taking them.

BARE BASICS

How to Spot Him

A jolt of energy hits you, and in a flash, a curious creature appears before you. He has shifty eyes and an overwhelming enthusiasm that makes him jabber on. You won't know if he is talking to you, at you, or through you, because his immediate and personal chatter seems oddly referential to your life, however uninvited. No matter, his ageless quality is charming and refreshing. He interestingly creates an inner debate on whether you love or hate him—because just like lightning, he strikes suddenly and fiercely, with odds to be awe-inspiring or devastatingly destructive. Oh Sagittarius man, he's so many things, too bad none of which includes having good timing.

In being such an unpredictable phenomenon, Sagittarius feeds off his instinct, sending him off at top speeds on "happy go lucky fly by the seat of his pants" missions into uncharted territory that touches everyone and anyone within his proximity. As a believer in volume, he's out to give a little piece of himself to everyone, so you can feel, ponder, and do whatever you want with it—no matter if you want it or not. He won't care who he offends either, covering the room with his rhetoric, because he knows the chances are in his favor of meeting at least one like-minded individual or an open apostle to click with his "turn your frown upside down" philosophies. Even if he doesn't, his optimism and persistence drives him to keep trying, as hope is his fuel.

It's this fearless attitude that makes Sagittarius sexy, as confidence and a positive attitude do that for a person. Just look around him, you'll notice his effect on people he travels with—and usually that'll include a large group of mixed individuals, all with interesting stories and a happy way about them, as if they all just stepped out of a cult meeting. But that's the Sagittarius' way. They are known for unifying the world in one happy bubble. If his aim is getting you into his crowd, then watch out, as he's a man that goes right for the kill. Not a guy to beat around the bush, his intentions are always quite clear. He says what he wants, when he wants, and in whatever way he wants. If you're making him hot and flustered, he'll tell you just that—and it might even slip out without him even catching it. His mouth often acts like a separate machine sourced out from his brain, churning out whatever is necessary to get his mind and body's desires into his clutches.

Although his blunt habit may get his foot caught in his mouth at times, it works well when's he out scouring the scene in search of love or lust, as there's no misinterpreting his intentions from him wanting a bit of you in his mouth. Then, if all is good to go and Mr. Magic Man is capturing your imagination and tickling your curiosities, get ready to batten down your hatches and blast off immediately into the passionate unknown, as Sagittarians don't believe in wasting time, least of all on anticipation.

Key Features:

♡ Big eyes that look as if they pop out of his head, constantly scanning where he is and where he's about to go

♡ A youthful appearance, either in fashion or physically
♡ A perpetually smiley face
♡ An eclectic and colorful style—traditional clothes/accessories
    from other countries
♡ Hangs with an international crowd and/or a wide variety of
    personalities
♡ Usually talks as if he's addressing a group or on camera
♡ A quick-paced walk filled with energy—always ready to go

Seducing Him into Your Boudoir

Sagittarians like getting to the point. If there's chemistry, it'll be obvious. His style is keeping honesty as the best policy, as being blunt
about who you are and what you feel is the hottest way to heat him
up. So, if he makes you sweat in a sexy kind of way, go balls to the
wall and let him know ASAP. With Sag, it's all about cutting to the
chase and saving the game playing for the bedroom.

However, while he's generous with giving out samples, getting a
more ample-sized serving can get a bit rocky, as consistency is his
problem. As nature would have it, Sagittarius is born with commitment issues, and as you get deeper involved, this problem gets
harder to maneuver around. As a free spirit, Sag is a man who likes
to play and that means playing with whomever and wherever. He
thrives on freedom and spontaneity, and connecting with mass amounts
of people. Yet despite it all, he's generally a believer in soul mates,
and at the end of the day all his carousing around is ultimately his
journey to find his spiritual mate who can take him to the next level
of love and understanding. Sure, it may take something short of a
miracle to get this stallion reined in, but this is the kind of love he
believes in. Until he finds that magic combo of depth, spirituality,
spontaneity, independence, and a never-ending listener to believe,
support, spread, and add to his rhetoric, he'll do as he pleases to
have himself a good ole time.

Obviously, being his soul mate is a non-negotiable position and he'll either feel it or not, but the qualities that make him wonder are your abilities to keep surprising and challenging him. After all, in taming him, one must be able to bring something into his life that he has never felt before—which can be opening him up to a religious ideal, cultural experience, or a philosophical system. He thinks he knows it all, so he yearns for a lover who is ten steps ahead of him, happily catching him off guard and providing him with all sorts of erotic explorations, risqué thoughts, and plain ole sweetness—and if you can wow him over and over again in this manner, then consider yourself a contender.

Loving Him in the Boudoir

Every day is sunny when you're with Sag. No matter what distress you may be facing, he always sees the silver lining and provides a positive outlook complete with a fantastical lesson with a happy ending—as that's the only kind he believes in. Sure, this fairy tale way of living isn't the most realistic, but he somehow always makes it work and usually lands on his feet. Of course, operating on such an idealistic level can make him be a disillusioned fool who never comes to terms with reality, but those Sags are apparent upon meeting, because there's always a 30 percent failure rate with Sag's optimism. Either or, he's always ready for good times.

As for how this attitude carries over in the boudoir, it makes Sag a good lay every time he hits the sack. His belief: All sex is good sex, and each time he unzips his pants to let loose his horny mongoose, it's as if each time is his first. Yes, no matter what comes his way, Sagittarius always make the most with what he's got, when he's got it, and he uses his imagination to go beyond, throwing in as many surprises as possible—like role-playing, edible treats, or anything he can integrate to make the experience as fun as possible. Of course, his aim at hand is orgasms for everyone, and his brass ring is making them as memorable as possible. Plus, as a physical creature, he'll work his body and yours until the last drop of sweat falls off your skin and the only thing left is sleep. So, if you rustle a Sag into your powers, be ready to work it like you've never worked it before and be able to dive into an adventure, because once he's given a task, his aim is to find the quickest and wildest route to a very fulfilling destination, making you swoon even if it's just from the sheer speed of it all.

MAKING HIM COME TO THE PALM OF YOUR HAND

Eye Candy

Sag men are more about checking out your body than your latest fashions. Clothes to him are like gift wrapping—a tease. To get him at maximum play mode, dress your package up as festively as possible, as this creates excitement. Think color, jingly accessories, and tons of panache, as his enthusiasm will equal a kid in a toy shop when you put on the bells and whistles. Be the epitome of fun, but keep him guessing, as he loves surprises. He lusts for spirited lovers, and if you've got that zing in your step, then your style should reflect that—international flair, self-made clothes, or anything that shows your independence and love of life—put it on and turn him out.

Stylin' Seduction:

♡ Lots of colors! Be wild and take chances, even if you look like a blind five-year-old orangutan dressed you. If you've got the spunk, he'll dig that. Just don't forget purple, his signature color.

♡ International styles, ethnic looks. He's a global traveler, if only in his mind—and being the sign most prone to date outside his race, religion, culture, etc., he'll love a worldly style.

- ♡ Athletic wear. Best to be comfortable and ready to go. You never know where you might wind up with this one.
- ♡ Plain jeans and T-shirt. He's a no-frills kind of guy, and if you can pull off casual au naturel, that's as hot as anything he could ask for.
- ♡ Trashy-chic. This look excites him, as long as you've got the class and wit to back yourself up.
- ♡ Flashy costumes. This guy lives his life as if he were on a float traveling down the main drag, so dress to join him.
- ♡ Accessories. It gives him more stuff to fiddle with and an excuse to get his paws on you.

Tasty Treats

Food

He'll put anything in his mouth, at least once, as Sag's list of life's "to-dos" is long, and the only way to ensure he'll get it all done is by indulging all his curiosities. He yearns to experience everything, as he's an adventure buff who loves a good adrenaline rush—the more exotic the better. So, in fueling his body, go off the beaten path to find what he hungers for. New cuisines, international fare, any spiritual or cultural rituals involving food or bizarre twists to the normal dining experience are all ways to score points, as the bragging rights alone will be delicious.

Erotic Eats:

- ♡ Medieval times. It's fun and it has horses—the favorite animal of Sagittarius.
- ♡ Dinner from a foreign land or religious rituals involving food. A place that provides him with a cultural experience will sound tasty to him.

♡ Sports bars that serve burgers. Sags have a no-frills hungry jock side that'll find this romantic.

♡ Restaurants that serve rare meats. Exotic kills excite him, as will the rush of newness.

♡ Alfresco dining. He's the outdoorsy sign, so this could be a picnic after a long hike to a fabulous summit or a rooftop BBQ.

♡ A casino restaurant. He's the sign of gambling and loves anything that's over the top.

♡ A dinner party. He's the date that'll do well around new people and will enjoy being your arm candy.

Movies

Sagittarians are always out for a good time, so forget trying to dull this vibe with serious cinema that can cause a downward spiral of emotions—unless the ending is inspiring. Not that he can't handle heartbreak, but paying admission to partake in something like that will seem utterly ridiculous to him. If he's going to have to sit still for two hours, he needs to be entertained, via humor, adventure, fantasy, or foreign intrigue. He needs to feel enlightened by philosophical or spiritual manifestos—as it's only the best of life for him or he's a no-go.

Cinematic Foreplay:

♡ Indie black comedy. Something smart and funny, just like him.

♡ Adventure. Ones based on extreme conditions and moral dilemmas are his favorites.

♡ Documentaries. Anything involving spirituality or is international will be superb.

♡ Movies with a spiritual plot, theme, or message in some form or another—something like *Baraka* or even the *Lady of Fatima*.

♡ Foreign flicks. We've gone over this a million times . . . He has a fetish for all things international.

♡ Cheery pop culture trash—his guilty pleasure. If anything, he's got to keep in touch with what the "regular" people are doing.

♡ Sci-fi or fantasy films. Movies loaded with special effects that teach a moral ideal are his thing.

Dating Ideas

Sagittarians are brewing with energy. Even though he also has the propensity to be a procrastinating couch potato, you can bet he's thinking of a zillion places while sitting in that one spot. However, most of the time you can count on him always being on the go. Sag lives to use every second of his day. In fact, it's Sag's goal to see and experience as much of the world as possible, even if it's on TV from his La-Z-Boy. Being that his curiosity is never ending, any adventure, new sport, or place he learns about is a challenge for him to experience and try to understand. If you'd like to play in his reindeer games, you need to be ready to journey to the edge of the universe and back because he dreams and plays big.

Playful Planning:

♡ Your house for a movie marathon. It's a great way to get him over to pounce on.

♡ Outdoor sports. From paintball to skydiving to river rafting to hang gliding to long bike rides, he'll do and love it all!

♡ A cultural activity. From a Japanese tea ceremony to a Trekkie convention, any kind of group that forms its own culture will be interesting to him.

♡ Horseback riding. All Sagittarians have cowboy fantasies. Another variation would be hitting the horse races. Sags love gambling, horses, and booze. Mix them together and get his perfect day.

♡ A religious event. Even if you both don't have a relationship to the event, he's always curious to see how others live and what they believe in.

♡ Karaoke. Rare is there a Sag who doesn't love it. They're the sign of the public speaker, so this goes hand in hand with his orator fantasies.

♡ A party. He's social and your relationship will be, too. Go and test your public chemistry. It'll intoxicate him to no end when you prove your public approval rate is high.

Sound Seduction

Conversation

"Why?" is the ultimate Sag question. He's inquisitive and out for the truth. He wants to know the meaning of life and the ins and outs of everything. Call it neurotic or curious, but this is how he deals. He yearns for spiritual expansion and a deeper self-awareness—as there's always room for improvement. However, this can make him get preachy. So, in conversations, be warned that sometimes he takes control and talks at you, instead of with you. Know you'll have to be able to keep up with his zeal to share your vast and passionate philosophical beliefs, spiritual understandings, and any form of truth you subscribe to, as that's what he'll be looking to uncover. If you can be funny all the while, no doubt he'll fall in love with you.

Icebreakers:

♡ Discuss the meaning of life. This is Sag's never-ending obsession.

♡ Ask him his religious/spiritual beliefs. What does he think happens after death? Learn how demented or brilliant he is.

♡ Bring up traveling and ask the most memorable places he's been to. Throw in a fantasy question for fun, too, like top five places he'd go to if money and time were no object.

♡ Have him describe the utopian society he'd want to live in. Sag has idealistic methods on running the world; he'll be thrilled to share them with you.

♡ Ask him about the most life-changing experience he's had so far. Be warned though, this is the guy that has an epiphany every other hour.

♡ Find out what he'd like his biggest contribution to the world to be. All Sagittarians have visions of grandeur. This is a good question to get out of the way fast, as you can gauge his disillusionment factor.

♡ Bring up past lives and see where he goes with it. Who he thinks he was. Whether he takes this seriously or comedically, he'll love imagining the possibilities.

Music

It's all about high energy with this uber-positive sign, so put on the tunes that can keep Sag's mood up. As you know, he's in search of the ultimate experiences in life. With music, he needs the same: something uplifting, which includes lyrics, music, and voice. Of course, you better not forget he's a fire sign, so he'll want intensity as part of the mix too, along with some spirituality and raw passion that'll get his body grooving and mind soaring to new heights of consciousness. In other words, use music like a drug. Think uppers all the way.

Mood Makers:

♡ Music from other countries or regions. For example: bhangra, samba, Dixieland, etc. Anything cultural turns him on.

♡ Pop music, as in Top 40 from any contemporary time frame. Pop culture is his guilty pleasure.

♡ Drum and bass. The beats will go right into his pants.
♡ Experimental music integrating bizarre musical instruments. He'll love the mind-expanding experience.
♡ Ballads, heavy metal, or pop. Sag likes anything he can belt it out with.
♡ Dance music. A party atmosphere is always good with him.
♡ Religious music. For example, spiritual chants, gospel, etc. This is the sign that rules religion.

Gifts

Sagittarius loves crap as much as the next person, but he's not material like his other fire-sign cronies are. To him, gifts aren't ego feeders, so price doesn't matter as much as its use, statement, and personality. He's way more into presents that offer memories to grow from than just possessing objects that clutter. Plus, since he's independent and impulsive, if he does crave something, he usually can't wait and just buys it for himself anyway. This then makes the trick of getting him something go beyond his need factor and straight into his want factor, as far as its conceptual and enlightening quotient. Yes, use your imagination to think of gifts that really do keep giving.

Boxed Treats:

♡ Spiritual gifts. Candles, incense, tarot cards, and self-help books will appease his inner spirit.
♡ A trip. Take him on an adventurous excursion—the farther away the better. He loves whipping out the passport.
♡ A class. Treat him to a language class, voice lessons, or any type of learning experience. With this gift, you can never go wrong.
♡ Throw him a party. He loves communal happiness.

♡ Camping equipment or sporting goods. Anything for the outdoors is fab.

♡ Things from other countries with some significant meaning. For example, a sweater from Ireland or a singing bowl from Tibet.

♡ A good watch. Not so much that he likes them as much as he needs one; punctuality isn't his thing.

Touch Me

Sagittarius vibrates on a level of perpetual horniness. In his constant search for nirvana, his body follows suit via orgasm. To balance his mind and body, he feels it necessary to satisfy both as frequently as possible. Plus, being a super-hyper spaz, he's got to take that energy somewhere and nothing is better than a romp in the sack to burn out the anxiety, transport himself into an alternate consciousness, and realign his chi. If this sounds like you, then consider yourself a match set. Just be sure you like it a bit rough and can work yourself down to the last drop each time because he doesn't like doing anything unless it's done to the max.

In being so idealistic, Sag expects a lot from his lovers. For one thing, he wants you to see sex as a necessity, like food or water. He wants you to approach it as if you've been stranded on an island deprived of it and gulp it down as savagely. He loves his sex raw, as that's your truth. You at your primal level is what he considers sexy. So be a beast and be all about the orgasm, as he loves cutting to the chase and being blunt with his desires. However, if you want to be the lover who scores extra credit, be able to discipline his animalistic ways by taking control and setting a pace that'll redefine his orgasm to be more than just a destination, but a result of a journey.

Besides being spontaneous and as bestial as possible, rope him in with adding more dimensions to the sex like tantric tricks, sex games or any kink factor you can throw in. Start slow, like doing

him in all sorts of locations, as he loves, loves, loves to mark the
world as his territory. Then move on with role-playing and sex exper-
iments. The point is to make Sag also use his mind during sex, challenging his performance to integrate all of himself. If he can burst out
an epiphany while he's at it, even better. He'll lust for you more. In
making him aware of you and how a physical connection of two
bodies in motion can lead to a spiritual union of orgasm, you'll be
talking his language. So, don't be scared to bring on as much freak-
iness as you can dream up, because he wants to show he's a cham-
pion. Yes, set those standards high and prove your notch is well
worth his talents.

Ways to Heat Up Your Sagittarius:

♡ Curl up to his hip area, his erogenous zone. Then lightly
   touch his pleasure trail, which can be found at his inner
   thighs. Stroke your fingers lightly on the inside and then run
   them up to his cock.

♡ Make your move somewhere random, as he loves sex in various locations. The more creative, the better. Although you
   can never miss with the great outdoors.

♡ Add a cultural theme to the erotic intrigue. For example: Dress
   up like a geisha or convert your bedroom into a Red Light
   district.

♡ Talk dirty to him in a foreign tongue or if you don't know any,
   take up an accent.

♡ Pick him up at the airport with nothing on but a trench coat
   and a sign with his name on it.

♡ Pop up unexpectedly for a quickie at any random place he
   may be, then leave right after. The flash sex will drive him
   wild for more.

♡ Take him to a sex club or party. He'll love checking out an
   alternative lifestyle, even if it's just to watch.

Role-playing

His brain has its own masterpiece theater going on—so in most cases you're already role-playing with Sag and you don't even know it. To get on the same page and add your thoughts in creating the ultimate kink fest, ask him to cue you in. Typically, he'll already have many plots created; all you'll have to do is choose a costume and scene, and add extra tension to play them out further. Scenarios he'll always opt for include anything fantastical, mystical, cultural, and cathartic.

Cast of Characters:

♡ Strangers killing time at an airport bar. Pretend you're both on two separate layovers, then wind up hooking up at a nearby hotel before departure. (Actually go to one and do it for maximum pleasure.) Anything involving travel or the idea of it appeals to him. His sign rules it.

♡ Nudists in the great outdoors. Being one with nature turns him on.

♡ Cowboy-themed fantasy. They all have cowboy fantasies.

♡ International pen pals finally meeting after years of sending dirty letters back and forth. Again, he loves anything that takes him out of his culture.

♡ A religious-themed fantasy. He's always looking for a catharsis.

♡ Adventure enthusiasts of some sort. Think explorers in the tundra in their tent after a day of fighting off the strongest forces of nature. Sag lives for extreme adventure.

♡ Cult leader and cult member. He's the sign most prone to self-help.

Taking the Bait

He wasn't born with a poker face. If he's happy with you, he'll keep responding. If unhappy, his mind will glaze over for a short period and then move on. He keeps a fast pace and is always moving toward the ultimate satisfaction. Sag doesn't do anything he doesn't like or want to; he's fiercely independent and worships his freedom. Not the guy to get tied down, he'll only stay somewhere if he wants to. Plus, he's immune to guilt and his blunt style doesn't make him the most polite either, so rest assure if your Sag is hanging around it's because he's digging you.

Of course, to tell the degree of how serious he is about you is another thing. It could be he just likes doing you or talking to you. However, if he can openly talk about the future with you, even if it's just tomorrow and having dinner, then take note: there's more to his feelings than just being your buddy—sex or otherwise. This is not the guy who likes to make plans, because his attitude is go with the flow—so know your eyebrow should be raised if he's ensuring time with you. The ultimate tip-off of his seriousness is if he wants to travel with you (if he pays for your ticket, too, even more serious!). However, only when you come back and can still stand each other, can you be sure that you're in. By venturing out into the world with him, it means something deep. His commitment must not feel heavy, but adventurous. If he achieves that vibe with you, then hoorah, consider yourself the daredevil genius he's been searching for.

UNAUTHORIZED: ASTRAL AUTOPSY

Recognizing Fear

Sag lives for hope and sees it as a happy and safe place where his imagination can be free. As long he's got it, he has something to strive for. Plus, he won't even need a lot of it either, because he knows how to stretch out his chances, and at the heart of it, he's got the soul of a gambler. Of course, there'll be those inevitable days when all goes bust and Sag's party crashes. Once in that pessimist pit, the fear sets in and the inescapable negative parts of life will then overwhelm, such as pain, anger, and confusion—all the things he normally thinks he has risen above.

Main cause

When reality blindsides him, knocking his rose-colored glasses off his face, fear is the time it takes to find those glasses again and restore his sense of optimism or the delusional sense of hope he lives in. However, this period is typically short because he aims to strive for an absolute happiness.

Immunizing His Fears:

- ♡ Keep a high code of morals and live by them. He'll feel safer being around someone with good karma.
- ♡ Believe in higher callings. He has a grand way of creating inspiration or delusions. Know how to talk to him, painting grand lessons he must learn and maintaining his indomitable "warrior" spirit.
- ♡ Keep a social scene rotating around him. He thrives in group situations.
- ♡ Forget time. The less restrictions he has, the calmer he'll feel.
- ♡ Always keep the lines of communication open. He needs to share his thoughts with you as he thinks them or else!

Infecting Him with Fear:

- ♡ Lack enthusiasm suddenly and he'll freak, thinking you're picking up some kind of negative energy.
- ♡ Constantly want one-on-one time with him. Sure, he loves private time with his Honey, but not 24-7. He'll get claustrophobic, thinking you're closing him in with neediness.

♡ Never have dreams to travel or at best, only want to go to domestic places. It's not that he'll be scared, more like he'll be scared of you.

♡ Make only one plan per day. Wasting time makes him anxious.

♡ Have him hang with a homogenous crowd and he'll be freaked, like he's in the Twilight Zone.

Recognizing Anger

Amid all his eccentric ideals is passion. After all, it has taken him a lifetime to achieve his wisdom and create a philosophical/spiritual practice to base his life on, making him fierce about his ideology. Never make the mistake of belittling them, no matter how off the wall or ridiculous those principles seem to you. The fact is his beliefs are his trophies gained after much introspection and suffering. If you dismiss them, it's like you're dismissing his pain. Any sideways remarks, condescending looks, or interrogation of any form will incite his mania, so avoid it all costs and save your laughing for behind his back.

Main cause
Offending his beliefs and making him feel threatened by an impending insanity.

Immunizing His Anger:

♡ Always be straightforward with him. The more direct you are, the better. He's all about truth straight up.

♡ Turn on the TV. Bright light distracts and quells any problem.

♡ Laugh. If there's a light way to deal, he'll always opt for that instead. Humor is always a ticket out of the murk known as anger.

♡ Change the subject by creating a fun diversion, like ask him to a movie. Spontaneity can easily erase any bad moment.

♡ Be happy 24-7 and live in la-la land—where anger doesn't exist. He'll gladly join you there.

Infecting Him with Anger:

♡ Be moody. Anything that distracts him from his happy-go-lucky life will annoy him.

♡ Infringe on his freedom. Stop by without calling. Spontaneity is nice, but only on his terms.

♡ Delay him. For example, park far away despite spaces close up or keep changing your outfit to avoid making it out swiftly. He can be late, but never you.

♡ Be aggressive about getting him to commit to plans at least a week in advance. He likes to fly by the seat of his pants; if you force him to do otherwise he may lose it.

♡ Distract his monologues with trite questions—like, "What do you want for dinner?" His words are important, hang on them or feel his wrath.

Recognizing Sadness

Sorrow is an emotion Sag looks to erase from his memory. He avoids it like the plague, as his attitude is that you can always rise above this base feeling and find an enlightening detour that leads back to happiness. If he does have to feel glum, he prefers it be as a compassionate experience. If it's an empathetic moment, he can deal, as this sends him on a mission to whip out all his uplifting words of wisdom and eradicate the melancholy for whomever the poor soul is. To Sag, sadness is a punishment and no one should ever get stuck in a condemnation like that.

Main cause
A weakness he must fight against.

Immunizing His Sadness:

♡ Need his words. Then, pop back to happiness after one of his pep talks. Believing he's got the answers to life will make him beyond happy.

♡ Never schedule anything early in the morning with him. Sleeping in thrills him.

♡ Give him some kind of religious or cultural amulet to ward off sadness.

♡ Let him know he inspires you. He lives to move people.

♡ Be excitable. Then, watch his enthusiasm come bounding out of him. He's very susceptible to feeding off your energy, but only if it's good.

Infecting Him with Sorrow:

♡ Be cautious and try to refrain him from his impulses. This could break his confidence, but only for a temporary period.

♡ Hide his good luck charm. They all think something higher is the explanation for it all.

♡ Throw back those blunt foot-in-the-mouth comments back at him. Rarely can Sag take a dose of his own medicine.

♡ Create a routine and expect a co-dependent relationship. This will sadden him for a little, but he'll solve it by dumping you.

♡ Don't laugh at his jokes. Dampen his aspiration to be the life of the party.

Recognizing Trust

If he likes you, he'll trust you. Even if he detects a few red flags (big or small), he'll edit them out in lieu of seeing you as perfect. Being that he's so independent, Sag isn't looking to trust people to, say, water his lawn while he's away or hide his secrets in. To him, trust is living up to his ideal of you. He gives trust out as endorsement. The more he likes you, the more hope he'll have in you and ultimately the more trust you'll get. Only when he feels you fall short and aren't living up to the stellar standard of life he's assigned you will his trust dissipate.

Main cause
Trust is the potential with which he has gauged you.

Immunizing His Trust:

- ♡ Be oblivious to the worst-case scenarios and be blindly optimistic—like him.
- ♡ Travel a lot and to places off the beaten path. Adventurous people mesmerize him.
- ♡ Be ambitious and have great follow-through. He'll trust who he admires.
- ♡ Know a lot of people and be well respected by many. Anyone with a cult status is cool with him.
- ♡ Have a grand explanation for life and live by your own ideals. Individuals with independence and eccentricity back his principles and are deemed trustworthy.

Infecting His Trust:

- ♡ Be negative. Expect the worst all the time. He'll think you're bad energy and won't trust being around you, as you'll pull in "sick" karma.
- ♡ Lack curiosities and live a routine. He feels regimented people lack judgment.
- ♡ Be anti-social. Anyone who closes himself off from the world has no sense of reality or truth in his eyes.
- ♡ Talk louder and prouder than him. How can he trust anyone who isn't listening to him?

♡ Explain yourself with too many words. He'll think you're being evasive and trying to hide something.

Recognizing Motivation

Sag can swing between frenzy and sedentary in two seconds flat. Always ready for action, he follows his impulses, which typically respond only to pleasure—including anything exciting, dangerous and/or possibly painful, as in the kind of pain that's a pathway to catharsis. He strives to be inspired and spread it around. To accomplish this, he lives life as fully as he's capable, going to the extremes with all his experiences and gaining as much wisdom as his mind will allow. While he knows being God isn't possible, being godlike is.

Main cause
Attaining his grand destiny takes work.

Immunizing His Motivation:

♡ Have no grand goal. Give him a situation where he's a cog and he'll eventually walk out.

♡ Bring him somewhere he needs to be silent. It'll drain him of his energy.

♡ Give him no recognition or audience. He'll see no point in being involved.

♡ Impose rules and regulations. It'll short him out.

♡ Surround him with low-energy people who don't like high-energy people.

Infecting Him with Motivation:

♡ Describe things in terms of a religious catharsis to jolt his curiosity. Inevitably he'll have to try out whatever that experience is.

♡ Engage him in daredevil activities and anything that involves adventure.

♡ Make it a bet. He loves to test the odds.

♡ Any place that possibly has a pulpit for him to spew his philosophies, count him in.

♡ Put a cultural spin to anything you want him in on. If he thinks he's learning and expanding his horizons, you won't be able to hold him back.

DESTINATION: DUMPSVILLE

Celestial Voodoo on You

Sag can disappear without a trace at a moment's notice, like an alien abduction. That's his style. If something better comes along, he'll just follow his instincts. In time, he may come around to tell you of his departure, but not without your putting his picture on milk cartons and worrying yourself gray. Plus it won't be like he'll have some grand explanation; he'll merely formalize your relationship's demise and disappear again. So, how to tell if you've got a Sag who's a loose cannon? If he's got the attention span of a gnat. This will be the type most likely to be a migrant lover, going where the opportunity takes him without even looking back, as he's obsessed with moving forward. In his mind, he'll ask himself if you're a part of his future, and if the answer is no, book closed. From there, he won't think about the past and least of all, you.

Sag thinks of himself as a constant flow of energy, and to avoid confrontation will think himself into believing he's powerless to how life plays out. If you have a problem with it, then that's your issue. He might even be obnoxious enough to tell you how to solve it, without recognizing his cause in your effect. To him, everything is done in the name of fun, so if you don't think so, he'll feel it's your responsibility to lighten up. In his world, pain, when felt by others, is an option.

. . . And Other Signs He Hates You

If an awful truth comes crashing down on Sag and he can't deflect it, expect his nasty side to come out. It's at that moment, you'll get why he has to do all that work to achieve a higher self, because his base self is such a bastard. For starters, his ego spits out fire, and once you challenge his peace of mind, he goes into his full-on competitor mode and is out to beat you at life. He'll do this by manifesting a dreadful fate for you, creating a story about how dark, depressing, and dreary your future will be, and how nothing good will ever happen to you again. Of course, it's pretty painless when it comes to your own existence, but if you believe in negative thoughts affecting your aura, then you're screwed. However, in the scheme of things, he'll pay the bigger price for the negative karma he's spreading—but in the face of hating you, he won't mind sacrificing some of his luck to ensure your suffering. No matter, in the end, this form of punishment will torture him more than anything, so sit back and take this opportunity to score your karmic points by hoping one day he'll find some form of spiritual guidance that can truly keep him intact.

Beating Him to the Punch

No matter how you dump him or how evil you can possibly get, you'll be no match for Sag's optimism. If he's into you, and that means way into you, he might not even register you've left or the agony you are actually imposing. He's so in his mind that he's generally oblivious to any form of devastating reality going on in the real world. To compensate for any possible injury, he'll create a happier ending to focus on and keep working toward that goal. This could even mean manifesting your return in his mind, which he'll gladly get lost in. In actuality, though, he might find it more satisfying than actually being with you because a fantasy means no hassles and a state of constant hopefulness.

Of course, it's not like he can't wake up from his goggle-eyed daze, but typically he takes so long to come to terms with misery that by the time it hits, his life has changed so drastically that he'll have new dramas to sort and create positive story lines for—and no doubt, you'll be long gone. If by chance he still has any residual disdain from you, he'll use it as a springboard to do more self-help work on himself and hope that karma will do his dirty work.

Ridding Yourself of Sagittarius with Minimal Scarring:

- ♡ Go on a major trip without him. It'll insult him and make him too jealous to deal.
- ♡ Hold him to his words, especially concerning time.
- ♡ Be devil's advocate to his ideas. He needs to have his dreams, even if they never come true.
- ♡ Be a homebody and never have aspirations to see the world.
- ♡ Be depressed and resistant to his pep talks. Whine as much as you can too. His optimism won't be able to withstand it.
- ♡ Tell him what he believes is cultish.
- ♡ Expect to have a private relationship. Close him out from the world like a kidnap victim.

Kick, Drop, and Kill

Sag's whirlwind love affair ends with a thud. Once it hits the ground, he's out of there and you're typically left lying there, feeling like Dorothy, but instead of landing in Oz, you're back in Kansas— back to a black-and-white world with definitive answers rather than high-flying ideals. Although you may be distressed to be in a lull after Sag's excitement, you have to remind yourself that although he might have been the captain on your adventures, you were indeed the co-pilot. You threw in just as much wild abandon to keep the pot brewing with thrills, and that part of you can live on forever. The difference with continuing your Sag-free journey, though, is you'll know how to ensure responsibilities to keep control, like paying attention to the details and avoiding the turbulence, safeguarding yourself from crash landings, which most likely with him were inevitable.

No matter, Sag is a fabulous treat to experience, like an all-inclusive cruise around the world. However, even with that, there's too much of a good thing as eventually that bloated feeling does take over, leaving you to wish you were home. Yes, exploring the universe and trying to figure out the mysteries of life are necessary to making it interesting, but knowing what's play work and real work is ultimately the puzzle we all must figure out—one he may or may not ever unravel. So, as you kiss your memories of Sag good-bye, be proud that you get the difference between being in the eye of the storm and being the storm.

WANTED: CAPRICORN

BORN: DECEMBER 22–JANUARY 20

A calculating and cold grumpus with a steely sex appeal that seeps out slowly behind his diabolical stare. Has a fondness for rules and regulations and will respond to the name Boss.

BARE BASICS

How to Spot Him

Capricorn emerged from the womb with a wise appearance, and throughout his life he has probably seemed more mature than his age would tell. With his serious demeanor and cool attitude, it's as if he's lived many lifetimes, all harder than the next and making him resilient to bullshit. Being a no-nonsense man, his way to draw in the lovers is always the same: The colder he stands, the hotter you get. Perhaps the truth is that he's really frozen in fear or it's sheer apathy, but it works and appears as if nothing breaks him. Just one look of his icy stare will do, possessing you like no other. His stance, his style, his habits, and his speech all ooze with a patriarchal power, irresistible for anyone with a bag load of father issues.

Winning the rep as the most anal-retentive member of the zodiac, Capricorn is indeed a tightwad and a control freak in constant need of rules and direction. He's the manager on jobs, the commander of order who revels in responsibility. However, there are other sides to him that only get revealed with time and experience. Like a bottle of scotch or a good cheese, Capricorn takes age to be perfected and an acquired tongue to appreciate it. If you have the patience and foresight to see past his rigidness, then enter at your own risk. He'll have a professional approach to strangers and prefers to keep quiet early on, letting you spill yourself out all over him. If he's impressed, then he'll make his moves. If not, he'll remain silent and keep watching you make an ass of yourself.

Not a man of too many words, unless necessary, his charm is debonair in an old-world kind of way. He's the guy to call to take care of business, get money advice from, and any other practical knowledge. The man that's good at all the seemingly dull stuff. Sure, he might not be as unpredictable and fun as others, but he takes things in differently, more methodically, thriving with discipline and structure. Having a good head for numbers, his logic and organizational skills often blind many from seeing beyond that. Most will underestimate his savvy, which is fine for him, as those judgments act like a filter to strain out the frivolous from getting in his way.

The ones who do make it through, though, may find a big surprise, as there are several degrees of Capricorn. While the most base level is the stingy miser who has crack-whore-bargain-basement hookers on speed dial, there are the precious few that are the esteemed unicorn Capricorns. According to the myth of Capricorn, while living on Mount Olympus, his original status was as a unicorn. Due to his greed, Zeus hurled him down to Earth and made him a goat. So, while many will have the goat qualities, there are some with a unicorn spirit resonating on a higher level than the material and are creative and angelic beings hidden under commoners' clothes. Which Capricorn you come into contact with is only detectable with time. In other words, don't let his ability to balance a checkbook fool you.

Key Features:

- ♡ Pointy or squinty eyes, chin, and/or face—a goatlike appearance
- ♡ Fine bone structure, a regal look to his stance
- ♡ A gentlemanly and/or patriarch look to him
- ♡ A soldier's gait
- ♡ Refined style—expensive labels and a polished look
- ♡ Dressed in office attire—professional looking
- ♡ One piece of flash to show off his status

Seducing Him into Your Boudoir

On the outside, Capricorn hardly looks like a freewheeling crazy sex machine. However, on the inside this guy is all kinds of kinky. Call it repression or a nice surprise, but if you want to get to the delicious nougat within, you're going to have to do the biting, as he's typically too polite for his own good. In doing so, approach the matters coolly and calmly, as he operates on a serious level and takes on the hunt like a business merger. He likes to acquire through hard work, preferring to gain affections with gentlemanly tactics. Take his lead and work your class with shrewdness, showing off your brains and ambition. Then, as soon as you know he's getting your vibe, flush those formalities down the drain and set the mood in motion by unveiling your perversions.

In a flash, Capricorn will go from staunch professor-type to revealing his true self: a horny goat out to graze all over you. After all, he's smart and doesn't take long to get a hint. He yearns for a lover that can be prim and proper on the outside, 100 percent nasty on the inside. By uncovering your sexy dominant side, he'll be all ears. Not to say he doesn't have the oomph to take you beyond missionary himself, it's just that he operates better being controlled and tends to get off better as the submissive. He'll want you to set the tone and define how freaky you want it to be. Then depending on how adaptable he is, he'll follow along. Add to his enthusiasm by being intrigued by his work. Pepper the chase with well-placed compliments on his attire, as he's always in need of approval.

Once you get him eating from your hands, let Capricorn know what it takes to win you. He loves structure and knowing the ladder of achievement he needs to climb to win your heart and is a quality worker all the way. In fact, any area you have him perform, he'll aim to get a gold star, as his goals are always about getting results. So, be exact in your demands and your bravado should pay off in a hot and steamy exchange that's sure to make Capricorn's stock rise.

Loving Him in the Boudoir

No matter what the task, Capricorn is so ambitious that he makes everything a competition. In the sack this works out beautifully, as he'll be a maniac to make you want him. Who cares what he needs or wants? He's so preoccupied with being good that it almost seems as if the affirmation is what gets him off. So, play the game by rattling off what makes you hot; he'll be more than happy to oblige your sexual to-do list. Once he knows your standards, all he'll want to do is take it higher and bring you where no man has gone before.

Who knew despite his anal tendencies that he could be a lover that can shock with furniture-flipping frenzied sex, if you're so inclined? Surprise, surprise, behind closed doors, Capricorn is a sexual beast. All you have to do is be serious about the sex and watch him go. He'll perform as if he's a part of an epic drama and do it with a dark and rough edge. He might even take you into full-out porn mode if you're willing. Dirty sex is his kind of sex, as it's typically devoid of emotion and all about skill—something he can perfect. Whatever kink you can think of, throw it in. He'll be a more than willing participant, as long as it's filthy and wrong.

Obviously, being good all day makes Capricorn want to be bad all night. It makes him a perfect lover for when you have lots of pent-up aggression. Enforce your rules and give him his due punishment: bound, gag, and flog him. He'll never get sick of being in trouble, as being controlled and obeying sexually excites him. Plus, getting feisty to overthrow your power is another trick he'll like to play. At the core of it, the mind fuck he ventures through is what sets the stage for his orgasm—so have your sadistic fun twisting him good. However, despite his abandon when action starts, he still is who he is and has a timer in his head. Meaning, start your sexcapades early in the night, as Capricorn still has to be at work in the morning, making his magic wand automatically turn back into pee pole sometime shortly after midnight.

MAKING HIM COME TO THE PALM OF YOUR HAND

Eye Candy

Capricorns are impressed with money. Reek of it and he'll be hungering for you like a dog at a dinner table. Although he might be a cheap bastard himself; he'd hate to look the part and least of all, hate to be going around town with dime-store arm candy. Look like you've spent a million bucks and dress to schmooze the world he aspires to be in. Just don't go overboard and get all flamboyant, as being loud is déclassé. Dress as if you're about to meet the queen of England and you'll be on his wavelength.

Stylin' Seduction:

♡ Simple and earthy colors. Black, white, browns, and navy blue are suited for his way of thinking.

♡ Labels. Money talks.

♡ Jewels. Status symbols make a look for Capricorn. The more expensive the value, the hotter he'll get. For fun, he'll figure out your tax returns as a married couple.

♡ Slutty and cheap, but only in private. Sleaze is his guilty pleasure.

♡ A business suit. He loves a regimented look or uniforms of any sort.

♡ Modest hemlines. A little teasing can go a long way.

♡ A nice belt. You never know when you're going to have to whip it off and flog him.

Tasty Treats

Food

Nothing tastes better than expensive. Who cares if he doesn't have the acquired tongue to appreciate the finer things in life? He's working on it, as he aspires to live the high life. Anything gourmet, trendy, or rare is what Capricorn craves. It's not so much about the taste, but about the psychological effects and to him, nothing tastes better than feeling as if he's a gentleman of the world. In actuality, though, most Capricorns would rather be home eating a frozen pizza, sacked out on his couch, and thinking about all the money he's saving—but when it comes to his image and trying to impress, it'll be necessary to go first class all the way.

Erotic Eats:

♡ Places with a historical significance. It could be a colonial restaurant where Thomas Jefferson ate or a restaurant where a mobster was shot—anything that has a story and history in it.

♡ Five-star restaurants with high prices and a kiss-ass staff. If you can make him feel important, he won't even care about the food.

♡ A restaurant with a minimalist design or a stylized look. When it comes to elegant atmospheres, Capricorn is less interested in the food and more focused on the ambiance and how cool he looks to be seen there.

♡ Steak houses. You can never go wrong with this, as it's a place a businessman would go to.

♡ Celebrity hot spots. Although he'll say he's above the whole pop culture thing, he does like to brag about places to be seen.

♡ Traditional dating places with candlelight and flowers. He's an old-fashioned guy at heart.

♡ An S-&-M-themed restaurant of any place with a staff decked out in leather. He's their niche customer.

Movies

The man is crazy about history. Capricorn loves archiving, being up on the news, and being part of significant moments that reflect the times. He's a never-ending source of information and fueled with all sorts of educational tidbits. Even seeing a movie will be serious for him because he'll want to learn something from it or be part of a cultural phenomena. Movies with critical acclaim or controversy are his preference or any form of cinematic brain food. Think of films he can discuss at a fancy dinner party and you're thinking like a Capricorn. Of course, if you wanted to drag him to see grossly obscene and totally trashy porno, well, as long as it's your idea, that'll be fine, too.

Cinematic Foreplay:

♡ Award-winning or critically acclaimed movies. He's all for a professional's opinion.

♡ Historical-themed films. They're perfect for his addiction.

♡ Epics. Movies that give him the most for his money.

- ♡ Documentaries. He appreciates any form of learning.
- ♡ Sex-filled erotic themes as long as It's not "silly." As a perv under a pin-striped suit, he'll love it.
- ♡ Sci-fi and fantasy flicks. Most Capricorns have a geek propensity, but not all of them are out with it.
- ♡ Black comedy. As long as it's twisted, as he's very comfortable laughing at others.

Dating Ideas

He's a toss-up kind of guy; open to suggestions and willing to bend anyway you want him to. At times, Capricorn can be so flexible that it may seem as if he has no personality. Being a solitary creature, he tends to be fairly rigid and sticks to his traditions. If you want to have fun or have an inkling of long-term interest in him, best to break him in and loosen him up with lighthearted and fun experiences. Once you get him cooking, he'll ease up and show that he can laugh and be a goofball, too. However, know that there's typically a little old man manning his controls, preferably driving him toward more urbane pursuits.

Playful Planning:

- ♡ Golf. It appeals to his inner gentleman.
- ♡ A cigar bar with a good stock of aged scotches. Anything old comforts him.
- ♡ Mountain hiking. He's symbolized by the mountain goat.
- ♡ A soccer match or paddleboat. Anything involving the calf muscle works for him—he rules that part of the body.
- ♡ Renting a status car. He'll love driving around so people can look at you.
- ♡ Trivia nights at a bar. Here he can flex his book smarts and nab a prize in front of an audience.

♡ An exclusive event. It could be anything, as long as the word "exclusive" is attached it to. Black-tie events for charity, even better. He loves social climbing!

Sound Seduction

Conversation

Capricorn loves to show off his knowledge as truth. Any topic you choose to discuss is fab, as long as it steers clear of imaginative or personal matters. Not comfortable with intimacy straight off, he needs to get tenderized first. The best way to soften him up is letting him rattle off his trivia on history, current events, financial affairs, and practical matters, or if he's the more progressive type, mystical matters. Then slowly ease him in by asking his advice on something personal to you. Being a natural fatherly type, he's typically wise beyond his years and can provide profound insights. To open this side of Capricorn, though, means first acknowledging his vast intellect with dry, yet deep, discussions.

Icebreakers:

♡ Find out the most expensive thing he has purchased. The first major purchase he made in his life? He'll love to brag about his splurges.

♡ Discuss his favorite book. Most Capricorns are fairly literary.

♡ Ask him about history. What events would he liked to have experienced? This can give you insight into his passions and depth.

♡ If he had a million tax-free dollars and only a week to spend it, what would he do with it? He loves talking about money, and this eases out his imaginative side.

♡ Bring up politics. Get this one over with right away, as this will be a major topic for him.

♡ Talk about his job. Why did he choose it and what does he love about it? Capricorns are work-a-holics and he loves talking about work, even if it's just bitching about it.

♡ Ask him about good investments. Even if you don't have the best chemistry with him it's always good to get something out of him. Sometimes money is better than sex.

Music

Like everything about him, he likes refinement. Capricorn loves his classics in whatever genre or subject you're talking about. As far as music goes, his tastes tend to be the tried and true, the masters, the originator of a genre, or the musicians that are at the top of their field with proof—such as a slew of famous fans that were inspired by them, record sales, awards, or any form of recognizable success. He likes to know his tastes are the best of the best, and this can spread into any category. Music that moves him is music that requires a skilled ear to appreciate. Yeah, you know it, he's totally pretentious.

Mood Makers:

♡ Classical. It's a solid choice to soothe him into your submission.

♡ Old jazz, blues, and/or soul. He relates to anything that draws inspiration from hard living.

♡ Drum and bass. Primal beats will appeal to the raw side of him.

♡ Folk/country. There's a crunchy/twangy edge to some Capricorns.

♡ Music from different time periods that capture a part of history. Again, he loves anything with a historical value.

♡ Songwriting musicians everyone looks up to. He likes to have educated tastes.

♡ Lounge. Music he can drink to and feel somewhat sophisticated with will bring out his suave side.

Gifts

Price matters and often if it's expensive it'll supercede any other aspect of the gift. No matter how useless or ugly it can be, if it's obviously costly, Capricorn will be completely impressed and find total affirmation through the money splurged. Of course, if you can think pricey and queue in further to his personality, appease him with anything that's practical. Items he can use at work are the most fitting, as he's a total work-a-holic. Even decor for his office will be superb, especially if it appreciates with age. The best presents for him are about needs—as in his need to be stinky rich or at least feel like it.

Boxed Treats:

- ♡ A wallet or a piggy bank. Anything money related works.
- ♡ Gift certificates. It's as good as money.
- ♡ Old coins or such. Anything he collects will definitely be something of value.
- ♡ A trip. He can always use one.
- ♡ History books, biographies, or memoirs. All topics he loves.
- ♡ Status accessories. Things like designer sunglasses or impressive cuff links—subtle forms of flash.
- ♡ A leather harness. So he never forgets who's the boss.

Touch Me

Sex is his necessity, like air, water, and earth, but this doesn't necessarily make Capricorn a passionately charged lover. No, he doesn't fuck from emotion, but from practicality and a primal need. Capricorn is more your man if you're athletic and want sex to be more of a workout than a human exchange. The truth is he makes love as if he's screwing a hooker. While this can be great for time management and generating a raw feel, he has a tendency to be clumsy and crass in the sack. To him, it's a euphuism for passionate and exhilarating, and if you don't care for him much, it's just disgusting — but take solace that he does get better with time and efforts. With any new lover, he goes through phases to learn your body and get you to learn his. So, expect infantile sex early on. Then, with a little coaxing and spanking of his ass, he'll fall in line and quite happily so.

As long as you don't drag in a ton of feelings in the early stages of your tryst, Capricorn will thrive and find his groove with practice. He's a quick learner and as long as you haven't cruelly badgered him about his lack of finesse, he'll be great. In fact, he loves a vocal lover who isn't scared to say what she wants and needs, but say it diplomatically. As you already know, he loves being controlled and whipped into submission. So, any filthy fantasies you have, lay them on the line. Once he sees your level of kink, he'll show you his — which you couldn't even imagine how demented it is, but yeah, he's nasty. Just listening to him will make you want to shower. However, only through journeying to his dark side of sexual secrets can you unlock his emotions, which tend to grow like fungus — taking time to germinate before taking over completely.

In allowing Capricorn to get into this compromising position and share the moment with you, it'll create a bond. After all, this is black-mail material and trusting you with it means allowing you to touch the deepest parts of him. So be bold and willing to go to the perverse parts of his mind, as this releases his magic within. Then, as your number of sexual expeditions escalates, know he'll start to reveal the "dirtiest" of his secrets, which is his tenderness — but only with time. Yes, like fine wine, Capricorn gets better with age.

Ways to Heat Up Your Capricorn:

- ♡ Run your fingers up and down his calves and lick his knees. Strange, yes, but guaranteed to work; his erogenous zones are the calves and knees.
- ♡ Do him on a bed of money.
- ♡ S&M always hits the spot, but make him beg first.
- ♡ Take him to an expensive hotel and do him like a hooker. He loves being treated like a sexual piece of meat.
- ♡ Blow him in public. The danger will make him feel bad-ass into his next lifetime.
- ♡ Schedule an appointment with him and then show up in your best getup and do him at the office. Work and sex, it couldn't get any hotter for him!
- ♡ Send him porn, either your own or ones that best describe your fantasies. He'll study them to get you off just the way you wish.

Role-playing

Loosen him up by dressing him up. Then let Capricorn escape in fantasies of the people he can't be in the daylight. It'll rock his world. This will include various types of characters, most stemming from the past and having a sense of discipline about them. Even if you're with a wild Capricorn who is uninhibited and over his material stage, he'll still have fantasies about power and domination. If you can add historical accuracy in it, it'll engage him even more. The smarter and darker your scene can get, the more intriguing his performance will be. In fact, the shock value alone might be enough to get him off.

Cast of Characters:

- ♡ Master and servant. It's a classic Capricorn fantasy.
- ♡ Farmer and farm animal. This can be before and after the slaughter, as anything twisted and taboo will feel extra-delicious to him.

- ♡ Two bank robbers post-heist. Anything involving money will get him off hard.
- ♡ Sleazy politician and blackmailer. He has a propensity to love politics.
- ♡ Movie producer and a casting couch prospect. Again, a variation on the power play.
- ♡ Banker and foreclosure victim. Power and cash, perfect together!
- ♡ Serial killer and prey. A demented domination fantasy that can also incorporate his high intellect.

Taking the Bait

He's a traditionalist and despite his non-emotional demeanor, Capricorn is a relationship guy. Thriving best in organized circumstances, having a steady relationship means having something he can build and work on—his favorite things to do. If you've spent more than forty-eight hours together, he most likely is already considering you his other half. Not to say anyone he screws can get this role, but mainly he's gunning for a commitment. He loves security, and any place he can find it he'll go for it. How serious he'll take your affair is another topic, though. Many times Capricorn will have a relationship just because that's what one does. Love won't be the issue. For that, there's a whole other set of complications that he'll have to work through.

To know if Capricorn's in love or even capable of it will be evident in how much he spends on you. Only when he's cuckoo for you will he crack open his wallet generously to shower you with extravagance, as he's typically a cheapskate. By making an investment in you, he's ensuring your value to him. The more cash he puts in, the more he feels. From there, he'll work it like he's starting a business, pulling out his blueprints and integrating you in them. Once in the plans, you're part of something bigger than just a couple—but a

Capricorn-run machine with timelines and goals. If he respects your ideas and lets you dictate how he spends his cash, then he's serious. He's a planner and if he's for real, he'll break out the talks and put his money where his mouth is.

His ultimate sign though is when you get the formal introduction to his family and he asks to meet yours. It won't matter if he hates his family, either; this is still a part of the deal he'll insist on. The more official the meeting, the more he's hooked. To Capricorn, this is all part of his emotional negotiations that needs to go on in his mind. Sure, it can get a bit too old fashioned for many, but to love him is to love the process he must go through to manage his reality and future. Completing these tasks one by one is just his way of laying down the road to be able to move forward and sign his heart on the dotted line.

UNAUTHORIZED: ASTRAL AUTOPSY

Recognizing Fear

Capricorn is crazy for security and organization. This is why he works hard and is so anal. He's always worried something is going to happen, but he also thinks work is God. Together, it all rolls into one perfect knot of tension that keeps him going without looking up. Who knows if this is what he likes or if he thinks this is just the way it has to be, he knows that without it, he could possibly unravel. He thrives with discipline, rules, and deadlines. Unwinding the structure is like unwinding his mind, which would equal complete chaos and a total Capricorn meltdown.

Main cause
Fear helps establish limits. Limits set structure. Structure equals peace.

Immunizing His Fears:

♡ Be caught clipping coupons; this will ease his mind that you're as economical as he.

♡ Be a lawyer or have the number of one on your speed dial. He's all about precautions.

♡ Work overtime and like it. Like-minded individuals ease his mind.

♡ When splitting a bill, work out the numbers to the exact penny. He respects precision.

♡ Own or talk about buying. This shows how practical and mature you are. Plus, anyone who understands equity is his kind of lover.

Infecting with Fear:

♡ When you know he's treating, order the most expensive thing on the menu. Splurging makes him nervous.

♡ When driving, tell him you think you just saw a cop. Authority freaks him out—even when he's doing nothing wrong.

♡ Pay your bills last minute and do it in front of him. Unpaid bills make him anxious.

♡ If you rent a car, refuse the insurance. Watch his knuckles turn white while you drive.

♡ Tell him you're going to throw him a surprise party, but it'll be when he least expects it. Although he'll secretly love it, the pressure of being in the spotlight will scare him. Of course, having this party is optional on your part as the threat is what's important.

Recognizing Anger

He can be stern, somber, and stodgy—and when push comes to shove, Capricorn gets aggressive, but rarely angry. Having a supernatural control on his feelings, losing it means a lack of discipline on his part and not being the authority figure he'd like to think he is. Ruled by his logic, anger is a feeling he'd like to believe could be tamed. Of course, when the pressure is on and he's up against a wall dealing with work or money-related issues, it's inevitable his high-strung nature can break apart.

Main cause
When aggression fails, anger picks up the slack.

Immunizing His Anger:

♡ Be well behaved in public. No slurping your soup, talking loud in movies or libraries, etc., or risk evoking his angry chaperone persona.

♡ Work out major compromises via a contract. Signed agreements soothe him.

♡ Don't be wasteful—like eat an apple to the core or wear socks until there are major holes in them. He's frugal to the bone and will feel more comfortable if you are, too.

♡ Polish his shoes or perform one act of humility if he ever gets mad at you. It'll cure all.

♡ Never plan anything by ear. Make a schedule and have deadlines.

Infecting with Anger:

♡ Overtip a waiter, cab driver, or a person in the service industry who's done an obvious poor job. Rewarding bad work will infuriate him insanely.

♡ When he makes a big purchase, say, an appliance, tell him you saw it somewhere else for much less after his cash-back return policy has expired.

♡ Tell him you'll call right back and take too long. His time is money, so he would like to think.

♡ Be inappropriate in front of his parents, like accidentally say something sexual. Around his parents, he has no sense of humor or forgiveness.

♡ Make more money than him or win more than him when you go to a casino or racetrack.

Recognizing Sadness

Tweaking out emotions from Capricorn isn't easy. He's not a great empathizer and avoids feelings as if they're a disease. His preference is to operate on autopilot and be programmed for production. Dwelling on any emotions, happy or sad, isn't his style. He'll shed a tear for things based on nostalgia and the past, but only once he's processed the situation fully and distanced himself far from it. As for his current frustrations, he'll repress them—which inevitably fuels him into staying too busy to feel—just the way he likes it.

Main cause
When busy doesn't cut it anymore.

Immunizing His Sadness:

♡ Have a future plan and goal. Treat your relationship like a company. He'll feel as happy and secure as a pea in a pod.

♡ Keep cool despite any stress. Avoid crying or having any kind of emotional breakdown, as it'll freak him out.

♡ Talk about money, as in saving, investing, and making more of it. Ambition makes him thrive.

♡ Hate his enemies as fiercely as he hates them. He loves feeling like a team against what he's conflicted by.

♡ Always notice when he makes a big purchase and reassure him that it's the top of the line. He pumps up his ego with material objects.

Infecting Him with Sorrow:

♡ Do something déclassé, like bring a box of wine to his house—or worse, to his parents or an uppity friend of his. He'll be sad to know he'll never want to call you again after you're both done finishing up the box.

♡ Give him a cheap birthday present. Even if that's all you can afford, it'll still upset him. What you spend is a direct correlation of what he'll assume you think he's worth.

♡ Ask about his childhood. Capricorns are all haunted by theirs. Dive in and find that sad memory that curses him.

♡ Avoid his help or advice; don't let him play his patriarchal role. He likes his lovers with a bit of co-dependence.

♡ Add a twist to his jokes to get him the bigger laughs. He knows he's not the funniest guy, but stealing his thunder effectively will make him feel extra-inadequate.

Recognizing Trust

Operating like a boss, he treats everyone like an equal opportunity employee, and only through time and evidence of your hard work does he give his seal of approval, via trust. He's a shrewd man who knows time is the only test that matters, and he's got the patience to properly assess your intelligence, punctuality, morality, and loyalty, and discern how you then use them in accordance with each other. In other words, your success equals his level of trustworthiness.

Main cause

Trust is a status symbol.

Immunizing His Trust:

♡ Be good with money and time. Be able to work numbers in your mind. A person good with numbers has a good sense of logic and this is where he first looks to see if he can trust you.

♡ Don't have a loud and flashy way about you in public. What he can't control, he won't trust.

♡ Have a profession of power and status, even if just on paper.

♡ If you need to borrow money and it's a random amount like $54.19, pay him back to the exact penny. Trust can only be given to those who are exact, not people who round off numbers. Of course, this should only happen once. If he expects you to pay him back to the penny each time, he's too cheap to be datable.

♡ Avoid changing your look; that shows how stable you are. The more you're the same; the more he can settle in.

Infecting His Trust:

♡ Play board games and prefer to make up your own rules. If you truly respect rules, you'd respect them 100 percent of the time. If you can't, he'll wonder what you're trying to hide.

♡ Always talk about relocating or do it often. Your unrest will scare him.

♡ Use up or tell him you've used up all your vacation and sick days by March. He won't like people who don't love work.

♡ Be a compulsive shopper, even though you suspect there could be a sale coming up shortly or that you could find it cheaper somewhere else. If you don't comparison shop, he'll consider you reckless.

♡ Be caught messing with his alarm clock and make him suspicious. This is one appliance of his you should never touch.

Recognizing Motivation

Capricorns love work. Without an agenda, he's clueless. He
doesn't know how to relax, but realize this is how he likes it. If you
want him, accept this fact. As the sign of the work-a-holic, he's
obsessed with getting ahead. He loves money and the things it
brings, such as security and status. When he's unable to feel himself
and really be in his own skin, money is his affirmation, validating his
ego, intelligence, and importance—all of which he thinks makes
him likable, which is in actuality the heart of his motivation. Yes, all
he really wants is to fit in or at least know he can buy himself in.

Main cause
Acceptance.

Immunizing His Motivation:

♡ Bring in chaos. He'll refuse to be part of anything that's not
managed in someway or another.
♡ Laugh a lot. Anything lacking a serious edge stunts him.
♡ Anything he's in involved with has to have an ending—as in
a prize or a goal. Without that carrot at the end of the stick,
he won't have a sense of direction or motivation.
♡ He never can say no to bargains—whatever you want, stress
a low cost or play up the deal part of the price.
♡ Give him lots of freedom and tell him to use his imagination.
It'll confuse him.

Infecting His Motivation:

♡ Go someplace together to experience something with a historical reference. Say you want to go on vacation to the Cayman Islands, talk about its past and lure his interest.

♡ Competition motivates Capricorn—the more heated the better.

♡ Anything that he has to strategize will interest him.

♡ Pay him and he'll do as you wish. Cold hard cash always speaks louder than words.

♡ Whatever the event or task you want him to do, subtly drop hints that it'll make him seem more sophisticated and wiser. Like if you want him to buy a certain pair of shoes, tell him he looks smart in them.

DESTINATION: DUMPSVILLE

Celestial Voodoo on You

Capricorn isn't spontaneous, so if you suspect trouble in paradise there's always ample time to let him down easy first. With his disdain for failure, he's slow to the draw, going down every avenue, ensuring there's no hope and that doom is inevitable. After all ground is covered, he'll tend to take the high road and responsibilities for his actions. No doubt, he'll give a proper and formal disseverment of your union, perhaps a humbling speech and a few good cheers for nostalgia's sake. Then, you can both go peacefully on your separate ways. Of course, this idyllic scenario is only going to happen if he's truly as "mature" as he claims.

If you suspect he's a poseur adult, then this will be the time to place your bets. Awkward with feelings and especially awful with sad ones, Capricorn has no sense of how to be comforting. When confronted in a situation like a breakup, he'll turn into a complete shit head: performing demented mathematical calculations, weigh-ing out time spent, significance of memories, and cash used. The lower you rank, the more sadistic he'll be—trying to recoup his expenses via torture. He won't let you go until he's ready, either, playing nice just enough for you to hang on. He figures, with nothing left to get out of you and deeming you a valueless piece of ass, he can do what he wants—building himself up by tearing you down. Yes, it's dreadfully evil, but that's who he can be, which most likely explains why his corresponding tarot card is the Devil. However, there'll be no sympathy with this one when it comes to the end.

. . . And Other Signs He Hates You

As Capricorn's enemy, he'll be out to demolish you in a full-out dec-laration of war. He loves power and lives to put people he hates in their place. He'll do it by competing with you in any area he can. It won't even matter if you care, because he's so consumed by his hate that he'll be single-minded. Expect him to find a new lover before you and act crazy in love, lavishing them with extravagant gifts and trying to rub in your face that you are missing out on so much. His whole front will be trying to prove how much better he is than you and without you. Obviously, these are all signs that he's feeling the hurt, but being that he's an emotional idiot, he can do what he wants. In actuality, his effort to prove his superiority is his therapy—and in time, it's effective, especially when you're nowhere to be found.

Beating Him to the Punch

Capricorn takes rejection well because he can keep a stiff upper lip and will refrain from having a breakdown where you can see it. As long as you're polite and fair in your approach, he'll oblige. He's such a trouper that his resolve can almost make you feel guilty. However, if you need to dig deep under his skin prior to dumping him, it's easy. He's so anal that driving him a little nuts can be fun for anyone with a sense of humor. Do things like be late, short out on cash, and be coy on making definitive decisions, or beat him at games and laugh all the while. Avoid being serious, but with the little things.

To further get your thrills, reduce Capricorn's pride in small increments over time by making him feel he has to earn your approval; but this will only work if you can hold back your emotions. Poo-poo his ideas, even if it's a place to have dinner. Casually insult the restaurant; say how it sucks and only poor losers dine there. He'll tend to feel bad instead of seeing you as unreasonable. He already gets off being a bottom, so he might not even recognize this as a problem, considering your happiness is part of his job. So, if you like being mean, this can be good times. Screw with him as long as it's convenient or until the power goes to your head.

Ridding Yourself of Capricorn with Minimal Scarring:

- ♡ Be untraditional in your approach to love—suggest an open relationship.
- ♡ Be slow to commit and have wishy-washy behavior.
- ♡ Tell him you're broke.
- ♡ Suggest to him you want to donate his money to charity and lots of it.
- ♡ Put him under a spotlight.
- ♡ Be spontaneous as often as possible.
- ♡ Don't plan well for a future and be reckless with cash.

Kick, Drop, and Kill

Like everything Capricorn does, your relationship's demise will be definitive. There'll be an end to an obvious beginning and middle, and you'll come to see that each of those phases held mapped-out expectations, strategies, and timelines. Obviously, if you met his relationship quota, or if he met yours, there would have been the next level. Instead, you come out of Capricorn's crash course in Successful Partnerships 101, learning the structural issues a relationship must face in order to work properly. It's a lesson that's invaluable in showing you a logistical equation for spending time, weighing out affections, and seeing potential for all future prospects.

Once completed, relationships will never be quite the same again, as you'll permanently have a better sense of responsibility. For one thing, you'll know that it takes more than chemistry to make a good thing last. While it might not be the most glamorous lesson to learn; it'll make you that much more aware of the components you'll need to build a strong foundation in your next tryst (and doubly with another Capricorn). So despite the sluggishness he might have caused, realize that in the bigger scheme of things he was most definitely a worthy investment that did give some returns, even if it was just a smidgen, as nobody ever gets out of a Capricorn relationship poorer than they got in.

WANTED: AQUARIUS

Friendly faced android excited by buttons and bright lights. Not necessarily operating in Earth's time zone or dimension, but will come back in time for dinner.

BARE BASICS

How to Spot Him

It's said that one out of ten people on Earth are not human, but some other life form. This could mean an alien, a ghost, an angel, or possibly an Aquarius. Sure, he'll look like a man, act like one, breathe like one, but there'll be something different and more eccentric about him. He's otherworldly, extraterrestrial, a genius ahead of his time, a man of the people, and/or a complete freak who is just too friendly and wacky to miss. Yes, he's many things, but mortal won't seem to be one of them.

For the unsuspecting stranger, he's the guy with the crowds swirling around him. Not that he's under the spotlight, he's without ego in that sense, but he's there serving as the connector. Being the guy who attracts all sorts of life forms, he's a crowd pleaser and has a way with bringing people together. While working a room, Aquarius has always got something interesting to say and will say it to everyone. Not overly shy, he gets around to meeting everyone, thriving on human rapport. Just wait your turn and he'll make his way over.

However, regardless of the throngs of people surrounding him, his aura will have a loner vibe that casts a distance. To some, this is sexy; to others, he's a science experiment in the making. The reason for the lab-rat behavior? It's because he's driven by his mind, which is always spinning with information and keeping him in his own world. Then, on top of that, he's got his randy and hard throbbing pisser that's always pestering him for attention. Between his dictating penis and an overactive mind, he's being pulled in two directions: instinct and intellect. This crosses his wires when he's out and about, which doesn't make him the smoothest operator when it comes to expressing his desires. In one instant, upon being turned-on, he'll pounce, be overly pushy, and/or act like a Neanderthal. In another moment, he can get all shaky and lose his articulateness. It's because he can feel his longing but won't understand how to process it. In too many cases, he tends to get nervous under pressure, missing the window of lusty opportunity and landing himself in the friendship zone. In fact, that's the astrological house he rules and oftentimes it's to his sexual detriment.

This is not to say Aquarius can't get laid, because he does—time and time again. How? He's smart and he's got bizarre talents that can strike the chord of other weirdos. So, if you're weird, super-weird, and got the ability to connect your mental and physical circuits in a way that can be slutty, smart, and strange, then pack your bags and be ready to fly back to outer space with this cosmic catch.

Key Features:

- ♡ Friendly and smiley face
- ♡ A plain look with one eccentric physical quality that's his signature—a certain accessory or style of clothes
- ♡ A tendency to be a bit overweight
- ♡ An intellectual quality about him, usually fairly articulate

♡ A connector, the one who knows everyone but isn't ruling the spotlight

♡ Is a pervert

♡ A hippie thing about him either by way of occupation or being passionately involved with some effort to make the world a better place—a humanitarian edge

Seducing Him into Your Boudoir

He's a total pervert, making him easy prey. Most anything turns him on, as long as you put in a little mental zing. This makes it simple if you're smart and have a sexy bravado that's fearless about expressing your desires. So, be assertive and imaginative, as he's strange and is used to that realm. In actuality, the fun fact about Aquarius is he can have sexual attractions to non-sexual things. He's so mentally in tune that he can easily sexualize anything. Sometimes, it's easier for him to deal with objects, as he can deconstruct the inanimate without question. Usually, he's so in his head that he's created a barrier between himself and the world, making him more comfortable dealing with groups over individuals. So, once sex and intimacy come into play, discomfort in his own skin can come out.

In the world of the hookup, this doesn't necessarily bode well for Aquarius, which is why he's the sign most prone to marrying young (and/or being addicted to porn). He's way into the companionship more than anything, feeling safer with friendship over sexual chemistry. So, if he's got a good time in you and thinks of you as his sexy little buddy, then you've got the winning combo that'll strike his fancy.

As for the actual dirty business, he's all about the kink and the mental aspects of sex. He's a bit of an android and emotions scare him. When it comes to love, it's almost as if it's a business transaction. While he'll have many romantic notions and ideas, understand the things he best deals with are concepts. Putting these concepts into play is another thing, though, as performance anxiety can run high. So approach the subject by taking him into submission, or ditch the drama and passion of the sex and go right in as if you're going on an amusement ride, because it's best to take a fun, easy-going, and experimental approach, as that'll register with him, sending a surge of electricity to all the right places.

Loving Him in the Boudoir

Aquarius will try anything in the sack, as he loves the word "experiment." He's into nontraditional ways of getting off and will go down any avenue—the dirtier the better. He loves breaking taboos and making up new ones. Aquarius wants to explore and have adventures that'll pique his mind into all sorts of new realms. He's not the most physical guy though, so his sex is usually not as rough or raunchy as he might lead you to believe. However, in some cases, he'll overcompensate by turning into a complete animal. What he might lack with technique, he makes up in creativity. Yes, it's the kink you pull out and the imagination you put in that will put him at his best.

So, go ahead and take sex into non-conforming and non-sexual places. Explore. He'll be your sexual Christopher Columbus, taking you to a new dimension of pleasure. Let him break out his toys and have his way, as he can turn anything into a sexually operational device that spins out hours of pleasure. Just be warned though, he might be more into playing with toys than you'd suspect, as he's a big time masturbator and his self-experiments have most likely included using non-human forms to get him off. His nature is to go off the beaten path, but as long as you're solidly in for the ride he won't forget to make the action for two. So, while others use primal instinct to do the do, this man strives to be more evolved by plugging himself into headier vibrations that'll pump him up to maximum capacity.

MAKING HIM COME TO THE
PALM OF YOUR HAND

Eye Candy

Aquarius is into innovative style and ingenuity that's got function—and that's with all things visual. With fashion, at best, he appreciates it as a form of textile architecture. In most cases, though, clothes are just a fact of life, and any way you dress will be fine with him. Hell, he's just excited to have a date and possibly a good grope. If your outfit provides him easy access, expect bells and whistles to go off in his head. Of course, if you showed up in a sultry Halloween costume, he'd be all over that too. It's about dressing to capture his imagination and make him think—as that's the way you want your Aquarius, always thinking.

Stylin' Seduction:

♡ Wacky color schemes. He loves lots of color. Of course, the one you can't forget is electric blue—his favorite.

♡ Earthy styles and organic fibers that are eco-friendly. He's the original peace, love, and happiness kind of guy.

♡ Clothes with a built-in function along with style. Anything with multipurpose.

♡ Fashion-forward. If it's innovative and eclectic, put it on.

♡ That whole hippie style/bohemian chic. An easygoing feel to your look.

♡ Skintight clothes. Vinyl and leather are his usual preferences, but if you have something more original, go for it!

♡ T-shirt or anything with a political slogan. Rebellion or positive statements toward humanity reflect his philosophies.

Tasty Treats

Food

His cherubic waistline will tell you how much Aquarius digs food. It's his sport of choice, as food is his body's data that makes it tick. It's his delicious escape that most other humans can understand and something he can share in. Food is best if it's a social event because it joins people together, which is completely up his alley. As for types of food, he likes it all—anything new or old, and he knows no limits. In fact, he likes being stuffed, as it makes him feel his humanness.

Erotic Eats:

- ♡ Fast Food. He loves trashy food like anyone, but he gets off on it. It's a guilty pleasure he revels in.
- ♡ Experimental cuisine of any sort, as in ingredients and tastes. He's a dining daredevil.
- ♡ A space age–themed restaurant, complete with a cosmic decor. Anything quirky and technological is his speed.
- ♡ A dinner party. He'll love meeting people.
- ♡ Minimalist design and architecturally beautiful environments that offer an experience beyond epicurean.
- ♡ Rich tastes and flavors that leave you feeling stuffed and comforted. Foods with gravies, heavy sauces, or cheese are his favorites. Chicken parmesan is an Aquarian favorite.
- ♡ Foreign delicacies of any sort and cultural learning experiences are always good.

Movies

Aquarius is a thinker. He loves letting his mind roam throughout time and space—and movies are an obvious way he can get lost outside himself. Themes can be anything, as long as it inspires ideas, has good character development, and brings him outside of his reality. New concepts in film or experimental ways to portray ideas will be high on his list, too. However, anything that's deemed smart is the prerequisite.

Cinematic Foreplay:

- ♡ Sci-fi and fantasy. *Star Wars* most likely changed his life and he probably owned its memorabilia or still has some.
- ♡ Indies. Anything left of center is targeted toward him.
- ♡ Documentaries on science, inventors, architects—and that realm. Again, more brain food.
- ♡ Films made with new technology. He's the sign of the future.
- ♡ Porn. He'll be ready to marry you if you suggest this one.
- ♡ Suspense, mystery, and horror. It sets his mind into action.
- ♡ Political-uprising movies. He's all about revolution.

Dating Ideas

Aquarius' perfect day is lounging in an armchair and zoning out via TV, music, video games, or any given electronic device. If he does like to tinker about, it's most likely wiring things together or fixing some form of electronic machinery. In other words, his mind is his greatest babysitter. While it's not the most social activity, he'll do well with you in a low-impact and mentally charged situation. So don't strain him and think intellectually stimulating with minimal effort.

Playful Planning:

- ♡ Museums. Best if it's a planetarium or science museum.
- ♡ Lectures of a famous intellectual of some sort. He aspires to be one.
- ♡ A protest or peace rally of any sort. He loves revolution.
- ♡ Music, especially if it's a festival, which is all about Aquarian energy.

- ♡ Fishing or bowling. Sports you don't need to be fit to do and allow lots of time to chat.
- ♡ A charity fund-raiser party. Partying for a cause will strike a chord with him. You can't go wrong with killing two birds with one stone . . . or something even like donating blood would be interestingly romantic to him.
- ♡ An afternoon at a video arcade. He's an addict!

Sound Seduction

Conversation

He's an expansive thinker and can have conversations about anything. You name it and he'll have a bizarre theory. Aquarius is unconventional and the sign of the innovator. He's way ahead of his time, sometimes so ahead that he comes across weird. Go conceptual; go political; go sci-fi—as long as it's a matter for the mind, he's been there, done that, and will take you there to go on and on about it.

Icebreakers:

- ♡ Ask him about his friendships. How long is his longest one? He's the ruler of friendship and most likely knows tons of people. Find out who's important and why; this person will have the most insight about him, outside of him.
- ♡ Talk about political beliefs, but in more of a theoretical way: his idea of a perfect society and how'd he run things. This will strike his humanitarian side—his passion.
- ♡ Bring up time travel. Does he believe in it? Where would he go? Back or forward? Why? He loves his sci-fi futuristic geek stuff.

💛 Ask him about the future: what he thinks the world will be like in a thousand years. Gauge if he's an optimist or a pessimist.

💛 Inquire about his invention ideas; he has tons. Ask him what invention he would have liked to invent. See how creative he really is.

💛 Ask him what current issues bug him the most? Idealism is his thing; therefore, reality has to suck.

💛 He's a techie. Ask if he thinks computers will replace humans? When? How far does he think technology can go? Get comfortable when you break out this conversation. He'll go on and on about this topic.

Music

He understands music in a completely different way than most people. To him, music is a mathematical equation that he can construct and deconstruct. Mozart was an Aquarian—so this should give you a hint on how Aquarius can translate the abstract quality of sound into passion and energy, despite how stoic he may come across. Listening to music for him would be the equivalent to reading a book for anyone else. It's mind-expanding. Most likely his tastes are for music that's somewhat technologically based, whether it's super-produced, made completely electronically, or totally left of center. Get this and you've got the frequency he'll easily tune into.

Mood Makers:

💛 Electronic and Industrial. Anything with a progressive edge will hit the right notes with him.

💛 Psychedelic, trance, or anything made for mind-altered states. He's all for tripping out.

💛 Music with political messages. He's the original humanitarian.

💛 Polka or bagpipe music. Anything with eclectic instruments will interest him.

- ♡ Freestyle jazz. Music with an unpredictable quality exemplifies his mind-set.
- ♡ Obscure underground bands that no one knows about, except him. He likes being the one who's listening to bands before their big break, as he's a forward thinker.
- ♡ Foreign pop music. There's always the inclination for him to like what's normal, but with a twist.

Gifts

Aquarius loves gadgets and little do-dads that he can fiddle around with to create bigger and better things. He's an inventor, always looking to create a more efficient and forward-moving world. If he could, he would rewire the planet and have everything run by one remote control. Give him something he can futz with and make him feel understood.

Boxed Treats:

- ♡ A pervy sex-related gift or a kinky pass card for him to do something to you that you'd normally be turned off by.
- ♡ A high-tech gadget that's the latest thing. Aquarius always wants to be first with the toys.
- ♡ Gift certificates to a record store. It's safe and never goes wrong.
- ♡ Porn . . . obvious.
- ♡ Junk food. He'll appreciate it better as a gift, like it's a "get out of jail free" card.
- ♡ Things related to video games. He can't get enough of them.
- ♡ Spy stuff, like a watch with several functions besides the obvious. The more functions, the happier he'll be.

Touch Me

Aquarius looks at everyone as a prospect, putting out his radar and seeing what electromagnetic waves come bouncing back to raise his curiosity. What he likes to pick up on tends to be nonconforming life forces. Not to say typical things won't turn him on. Of course, he likes a sculpted body, a sparkling mind, and out-of-the-world charisma, but it's not necessary. Usually what rings his lust-o-meter at the top bell is a unique feature that tends to be somewhat odd, like a peg leg or something subtle, like a scar or even a strange ability such as being able to spin plates while riding a bike. He's a quirky turkey and his idea of a sex kitten doesn't necessarily fit society's.

Most likely because he feels out of place, Aquarius seeks out others whom he thinks might have a sense of exclusion, too. So don't be shy about sharing your strange and bizarre self with this nutcase. He's yearning to find a fellow freak to party his body. With an eccentric lover, he's gambling on having "off-road" sex. Understand he's a bit removed from his physicality, making the kink factor important, if not necessary. His lovers aren't afraid to be dirty and explore taboos. The sex he craves is unique and, at the heart of it, a bit perverted—because that's how he fantasizes about it. He's usually spent countless hours masturbating and thinking about sex in all different ways and with objects no one else would ever associate with sex. So share your strange tastes and he'll share his, giving you both a passport to a very seductively odd and devilish universe in which you learn there's more to desire than just doing it.

Once roped in by the kinky mind-fuck, make your sex as daring, bold, and experimental as possible. Make him your slave. In fact, that's really what he's after: getting someone to use him as if he were an object. Think of him like a sex machine and you've got the idea. Sex for him is like launching a rocket: Heat up the pad, pull back the ejector, and shoot for the stars. Master this and get your Aquarius on a leash, always ready to go home.

Ways to Heat Up Your Aquarius:

♡ In keeping with his oddball theme, his erogenous zone is in his shins and ankles. Massage them as if they're an extra-large member.

♡ Talk openly about sex. Be at ease to share all you've done and elude to what you want to do.

♡ Let him live out his hooker fantasies. Do him in a sleazy motel and have him pay for your services.

♡ Send him sexy photos and messages to his phone and/or computer.

♡ Whip out toys and mix other kinky items into your sex.

♡ Surprise him with guest "stars." He's a total people person.

♡ Pull out the porn. Merge the best of both worlds, as he spends much time debating which is better. With porn, you don't have to worry about emotions, but it can't spoon you.

Role-playing

He's up for anything that transports his mind elsewhere. Add sex to the program and there's no stopping him from going right into character. As long as it's bizarre, original, possibly technologically intriguing, and mentally riveting he'll give it his 110 percent. Expect the heightened senses of Aquarius in full attention, too, as he's all about team efforts and making a happy and peaceful world for one and all. If it means he might have to wear a silly hat to make it happen, then so be it.

Cast of Characters:

♡ Inventor of a time machine with a robot assistant. Choose to journey to another time or do it right in your machine, as anything to do with time travel will appeal to him.

♡ Two extraterrestrials. Aliens turn him on.

♡ Phone sex operator and caller. Remain in two different rooms and talk each other through a masturbatory exchange until each of you gets the other off. The idea of mutual masturbation turns him on.

♡ Scientist with defrosted cave person. Anything dealing with science or technology works with him.

♡ Futuristic humans. He's already a forward-thinking guy, so bring this into the sack and light up his life on several levels.

♡ Two computer whizzes trying to decode a program before a bomb detonates. Get the program figured out and save the world as the countdown begins. Then, of course, indulge in the victory screw. This type of pressure will build him up into a lovely climax.

♡ A *Star Wars* fantasy. You bet this guy will love to dress up like someone in the Rebellion and go for broke defending the galaxy.

Taking the Bait

Aquarius is looking for a fuckable best friend. His approach toward relationships centers on companionship, with sex playing a supporting role. He'll sleep around because he's a slut, but who he takes into his life as partner is someone who must be able to hang with him and his posse. While he'll have no problems being friendly and inviting to everyone, only the special ones see his private side and a role as his confidante.

To know where you are without a doubt, there's one place you can look for 100 percent reassurance—his friends. They're his board of directors, and only when you pass through their judgment does he safely give himself over. Yes, even despite all the kinky love you may give or how demented or deformed you may be, his friends must be won over by your heart. With them, he'll share his feelings and thoughts, as they're his biggest cheerleaders. If they take all the evidence and give you the green light, consider yourself part of the team.

As for commitment, it's a gradual process that won't necessarily get discussed much. He prefers a seamless transition, and a growing partnership. However, once he does know where he's going, he falls into line pretty quickly. The fact is that this man is a server. Since he's not emotionally driven, he's awkward with them and he'll prefer playing the part of pleaser (who knows if it's passive aggressive behavior, but yeah, he's easily whipped). At first, he'll perform sweet gestures in hopes of making you happier, then after a while he'll program himself to suit your needs, giving you a custom-built lover to do as you say and want. In the end, he's open with his time, talents, and any emotion he can muster up, leaving it up to you whether you'll want to keep the model or send it back—satisfaction not always guaranteed.

UNAUTHORIZED: ASTRAL AUTOPSY

Recognizing Fear

Aquarius is stubborn and doesn't like changing himself, even though he's obsessed with the world around him changing. Of course, it's inevitable he must surrender at the emotional crossroads, which is his most fearful situation. Yes, being human can be quite trifling and scary. At the heart of the matter, he'll avoid it at all costs.

Main cause
Realizing he's just a mortal.

Immunizing His Fears:

♡ Make him your robot and watch him thrive. Always have a list of things he can do around your house, like wire your entertainment system, reinstall your computer, or fix your car.

- ♡ Be pro-technology and future-forward thinking. Score extra points if you're on the same operating system as him.
- ♡ Avoid emotional breakdowns and keep things on a mental and intellectual level.
- ♡ Always put your extra change in the charity bins by the grocery's registers. Your humanitarian spirit will let him know he's in good hands with you.
- ♡ Tell him you were a dork in high school; this will comfort him like you wouldn't believe!

Infecting with Fear:

- ♡ Close him out from his friends; leave him to make decisions by himself. He's an all for one and one for all kind of guy.
- ♡ Push him to be macho; go to the gym and get him in the weight room. He's not one to be in touch with his physicality or his machismo.
- ♡ Be needy and want to spend every second with him. If anyone needs space, it's this one.
- ♡ Bring him around your most bombastic friend you know he'd hate. Being that he rules the house of friends, he'll feel trepidation about speaking up and offending you.
- ♡ Make him watch your favorite tearjerker movie with you. Emotions cause him discomfort.

Recognizing Anger

He's angry. However, anger at individuals is not something he easily deals with, not like being mad at a concept or an ideology. He revels in getting irate at situations, then spring-boarding into action. When anger challenges his idealism, he deals by facing up to his hopes that Utopia can exist. From here, he'll think he can change people, but of course, that's the hardest of all things to change.

Once seeing people don't change, he'll get angry again. It's a vicious cycle, but through the repetition he hopes something will give.

Main cause
Pain for progress, as he believes that's the price he must pay.

Immunizing His Anger:

- ♡ Be aware of the political climate going on throughout the world. Ignorance is not his form of bliss. He'll respect you more for being a thoughtful and conscientious member of society.
- ♡ Avoid being aggressive with him in general. It'll solve nothing.
- ♡ Settle any disputes by taking him out to dinner. Food can always be your white flag.
- ♡ Always include his friends. He's about creating and being part of a community.
- ♡ Appreciate his eccentric behavior and be bizarre with him. Love going to *Star Trek* conventions, quote *Star Wars* movies, etc.

Infecting Him with Anger:

- ♡ Get your news from tabloid magazines or non-news TV shows. He'll dump you in time, but not without being pissed off about your consumer mentality.
- ♡ Buy plastic utensils and non-recyclable products whenever you're with him. Never throw your garbage out in proper bins. Be un-PC.
- ♡ Make racist or classist jokes in jest. He will fail to see the humor and find you offensive for thinking it is.
- ♡ Cut in lines and think of yourself first, always.
- ♡ Use his computer or trinkets without asking. He's precious about them and likes to supervise anyone going near his electronic gadgets.

Recognizing Sadness

He suffers from a chronic case of cynicism that makes him feel like a perpetually misunderstood intellectual. His intelligence is his pain, a thorn in his side, and for that, there's always an excruciating awareness of the isolation and loneliness of his existence. Yes, it's a mournful situation to be so ahead of one's time.

Main cause
It's his burden to be so brilliant; his depth is a loneliness that he must bear.

Immunizing His Sadness:

- ♡ Distract with perversion. He's always happily sidetracked by anything dirty—and that's perverted, not necessarily sexy.
- ♡ Ask him about politics and progressive ideals. Treat him as if he's an intellectual.
- ♡ Let him have control of the radio in the car or choose the restaurants you go to. It's letting him have control over the little things that'll please him.
- ♡ Laugh at his jokes, despite his miserable delivery.
- ♡ Always have a project he could be working on or something to fix. Anything dealing with electricity is best suited for him.

Infecting Him with Sorrow:

- ♡ Rig an IQ test and have it somehow give him a low score.
- ♡ Tell him a new model just came out after he just bought the latest tech-gadget.
- ♡ Call him a nerd, dweeb, geek, or anything of such descriptions. Even as a joke, it'll hit too close to home.
- ♡ Ask someone else to fix your computer.

♡ Send him tons of e-mail chain letters. Everybody hates them, but he'll go nuts being caught in between superstition and aggravation. Either/or, it'll upset him.

Recognizing Trust

Trust is a prize given to only a few. Applicants must pass through a series of tests, unbeknown to them, as it's not easy to get close to Aquarius. Being distant helps him maintain his idealism, so he's careful with whom he lets in. Being aware of how moral/immoral and dumb people are, he doesn't like wasting precious time with them. While he could put on a happy face for many, only a few will be awarded his trust, and only through the test of time will they know what that means.

Main cause

He needs comrades against a cold and heartless world who see life in the same way and wants to ensure the same standard of morals.

Immunizing His Trust:

♡ Be a Good Samaritan and have causes that you can support.

♡ Be nice to cabbies and waitstaff, and treat all people equally.

♡ Have high SAT scores, a high IQ, or be a part of MENSA. If you graduated from a top accredited college and were the valedictorian, share that info. He admires intelligence in the traditional sense.

♡ Be willing to share your ATM or computer password.

♡ Be able to have many friendships with all sorts of unique characters. He believes very much in the birds-of-a-feather concept.

Infecting His Trust:

- ♡ Be fearful of technology and "progress." He won't trust your backward way of thinking.
- ♡ Be wasteful and un PC. Be unaware of environmental issues, social dilemmas, etc.
- ♡ Feel competitive with his friends and make him feel as if he has to choose you over them.
- ♡ Be happy and not give into his attitude of cynicism equaling intelligence.
- ♡ Be money hungry. Nothing says "corrupt character" better than being a materialistic and total capitalist consumer pig!

Recognizing Motivation

Future-forward is his attitude and he's all about progress, but what's ironic is his belief/interest in technology has everything to do with wanting something to pick up his slack. Not that he doesn't love to keep busy for the sake of being busy, but he's motivated by touching anything with knobs, buttons, click wheels, pedals, wires, plugs, and everything of that nature. His ultimate wish: control of the world from a La-Z-Boy with a push of a button.

Main cause
He loves busy work and thinking of life as a giant science project.

Immunizing His Motivation:

- ♡ Don't approach matters with a dictator's attitude. He'll only respond well to communist methods.
- ♡ TV hypnotizes him or any flashing bright lights. Put them on and he'll submit.

♡ Play to his absent-minded-professor mentality. If he's about to do something you don't want, just sidetrack him with asking another random and detailed question.

♡ Bring emotions onto the scene and he won't know which way is up or down. He's best with moral dilemmas, not ones dealing with feelings. The more intense, the more effective.

♡ Require him to do anything physical and he'll lose his drive. He's mentally motivated, not physically.

Infecting Him with Motivation:

♡ Inspire him with activities that defy convention. Talk up any bizarre place and he'll be one happy camper wanting to go there.

♡ Appeal to his humanitarian sign. Nothing says "go" to Aquarius than nonprofit, volunteer work, and charity.

♡ Try anything that deals with future-forward thinking and he's in.

♡ Have a group project ready. Teamwork makes him thrive, especially if it deals with politics. He's all for starting a revolution.

♡ Any task that needs an intellectual solution will have his name to it.

DESTINATION: DUMPSVILLE

Celestial Voodoo on You

Aquarians are amicable. He strives for peace and that includes a world where he and his exes can co-exist harmoniously. His tact is tops and he's usually motivated to do the right thing. This makes him a gem in the breakup world, as he aims for an objective and pain-free solution. Being a normally aloof gent, he hates getting caught up in emotions, and keeping a cool head is how he copes. His Ideal Is to preserve some form of friendship, as he's opened himself up in some way and that'll mean something to him.

With his romantic entanglements mostly being based on companionship, he can usually switch gears into platonic mode easier than most. It's his talent to come across asexual at the drop of a hat and do whatever he can mentally do to avoid distress. In the end, his diplomacy is like that of a UN official, and he severs ties only after much talking, understanding, and compromising. Anyone would be a fool not to accept the olive branch, for obvious reasons. If you refuse, understand his psyche beyond this realm is not chartable and there's no telling what he might do if you don't resolve this situation in a controlled manner. Everyone has a psycho side, and this guy works on programming it out of his system. However, nothing is ever guaranteed, so realize when he's being gallant, he's being sincere and you should graciously submit to his request.

. . . And Other Signs He Hates You

Aquarius' high IQ can give him a high score in the asshole quotient too. Just as he can use his brain to create Utopia, he can use it to make hell. Being so detached and aloof, he's unaware of the intensity of pain he can inflict. So beware, in the face of hate, his dark side will take the reins and turn him into a sinister and cold anguish alchemist who won't recognize limits.

With enemies, Aquarius has no rules and plays it by ear. He'll act out cruelly in any way that can soothe his mind. At the least, expect to be sealed off from his circle of friends, as they'll think of you as a Satan, too. In fact, he'll make public all your ugly sides, but explained very succinctly. He won't be open about it, either; as he'll have a way of getting people to ask him and seemingly coax it out of him— but that's how he plans it. This absolves him of karmic payback, as he'll feel sharing his perspective on you is part of his mission. To him, informing the world of his knowledge is what he does, and if he sees you are the bad apple in the cog of humanity, he'll do what he can to repel you from its system. He's stubborn, so he rarely offers forgiveness—but make no mistake, he'll only pull out this behavior when really called for. It's not in his character to spread negativity, so know if he's gone there, you were the co-pilot. So be ready to face your karma.

Beating Him to the Punch

Despite his utopian ideals for humanity, he tends to have a negative outlook of his own outcome. Yes, most Aquarians have self-esteem issues and are prepared for the worst. This makes it easy for you, as it won't be too hard for him to sense the end. His mind is future forward and most likely has already come up with his own ideas of how, when, and where you'll dump him. You won't be able to shock him and he'll take his pain like a champ.

In most cases, the only challenge you will have is getting him to understand why. Since most relationships end because of something emotionally based, Aquarius will have a harder time comprehending the matters at hand. Remember, he's not emotionally wired, so you must be intellectual about information. Be straight about breaking up, give your reasons a conceptual twist, and be simple in your logic. Use the same approach you might use for returning a shirt that's not your size, because making it mechanical is the one way that the understanding can sink into his bones. He's programmed to please, so if you can get this process down, you'll be in the free and clear. In Aquarian terms, just go to his mainframe and detour his connection to you by providing another adapter that reprograms his circuits. Once you get the coding right, reboot the operating system and he should be virus-free.

Ridding Yourself of Aquarius with Minimal Scarring:

- ♡ Be frank and say that you can still be friends straight off.
- ♡ Demand he start exercising daily with you.
- ♡ Ask other people to do your handiwork and disregard the talents he prides himself on.
- ♡ Remain detached with his friends—not want to meet them, but not let it be that obvious. Then try to control him to be with you all the time.
- ♡ Be uncaring toward society or environmental issues.
- ♡ Be anti-technology.
- ♡ Hint to his friends that you're thinking of breaking up. Word will get back to him quick enough.

Kick, Drop, and Kill

Expect to decompress after being transported back from Aquarius land. With your brain all jumbled, it'll take time to reconnect with a recognizable and definitive sense of reason. Think of it like a major case of jet lag: you're disorientated, you know something out of the ordinary has happened—and just like any trip, there'll be souvenirs as evidence, such as your entertainment system working with only one remote, the clock set on your DVR or a pile of books on quantum physics in your bathroom.

Upon absorbing the memories and coming back into your own reality, it'll feel as if you spent time with an extraterrestrial—and perhaps you did. You might never know the difference and it can keep you pondering. With such a captivating mind, it makes Aquarius hard to forget. Be thankful, too, as it could have been worse. Be glad that he's not so much a jerk, as he is off center. He'd be great for another of his species and dimension. Who knows? If it were another time for you, perhaps it could have been great too, like when you're in an old-age home. By then, you'd have the patience for his bizarre energy and the space to listen to his winsome and weird babbling. Plus, he'd probably have a bit of sauce still left in him with tons more perversion to explore. Yeah, guess the problem with him is that he's just too ahead of his time.

WANTED: PISCES

BORN: FEBRUARY 21—MARCH 20

Pretty boy with a penchant for self-destructive nirvana. Beware, he can play victim at will; be cautious when you submit your defenses and cash.

BARE BASICS

How to Spot Him

To the untrained eye, Pisces can look oh-so delicate; making it hard for you to believe he can be left alone without an electric fence, bodyguards, and a security dog to protect him from all the perverts and scoundrels scouring the streets in search of innocent prey to defile. His harmless demeanor, his hint of vulnerability, and his heartfelt manners would have even the shrewdest person assuming he could do no wrong. After all, how could someone that can instantly understand your soul be bad? It would seem almost impossible to comprehend.

The joke is on you, if you're one of those marauders to spot this sweet and seemingly fragile being known as Pisces, who's really a master of disguises. His gentle creature façade that oozes of a need to be nursed is really just a guise to source out the suckers. Call it a protection mechanism or a villainous sixth sense, but with this man you never know who's going to pop up. He's an emotional sponge, and depending on his mood and how he absorbs and processes you through his feelers, you never know which side of Pisces you will tango with until sometimes it's too late. If his sensors are flashing green and he can't stop himself from wanting to wrap himself in your aura, then prepare to be shown the Devil in him and for a dramatic and passionate love story to unfold.

Yes, Pisces is that pretty boy who can make you fall in love with him at first sight. Of course, with his sensibility he's also looking to swoon at first glance too, as he's a full-fledged addict to romance, especially the theatrical kind. With him, he lives at the extremes and loves this way, too. It's his belief that he must go to the farthest reaches to be able to comprehend the range of emotions life has to offer. This could mean being a complete alcoholic or a devout member of a spiritual practice—and note, he'll have a propensity to be at those two extremes, too.

Either or, Pisces is a man with an infallible magnetism that he uses like a gypsy mind-reading trick, honing in on your psyche to conjure any number of emotions he chooses. In the world of the hookup, this power comes in quite handy in charming the pants off his prospects. With his magical way, he'll connect with you and make you feel as if you've known him forever. Once this bond is created, the possibilities will be endless—and if this can happen within an hour of meeting him, even better. Being the ultimate sucker for love, Pisces has no qualms in offering his heart immediately, as his instincts drive him. Besides, jumping in is the only way he can ensure a captivating quality to his love affairs, making fairy tales seem dull in comparison. Give him what he wants, by proving you've got the imagination and balls to dive right in, taking him on as your Prince Charming and beginning your happily-ever-after ASAP.

Key Features:

♡ Long eyelashes
♡ Typically slender with lanky build

♡ A wise and calm vibe to him
♡ A feminine quality, by way of prettiness or sensitivity
♡ An innocence aura that make you want to do things for him
♡ Prone to wearing a good luck talisman or some kind of spiritual charm
♡ Too much cologne or some type of strong scent

Seducing Him into Your Boudoir

If you can read minds, this is a talent that can get you any Pisces, anytime. First impressions are his only impressions, as he operates on pure intuition. It won't matter if you pretend a little either, as long as you put out sincere efforts—he'll adore you for it. He's sensitive to a fault and if you feel the slightest inkling of affection for him, he'll instantly have an endearment toward you.

Although, as the sign most prone to charity fucking, you'll have to tread lightly in figuring out how much Pisces likes you or is into the idea of you liking him. Since he gets off on indulging his self-sacrificing ways, use your best judgment to see if he's feeding his ego through you. If he is, then he'll get demanding, expecting you to pay for his time by worshipping him via cash, subservience, or whatever perks you offer. Assuming you're well adjusted, the way to seduce Pisces properly is by wearing your heart on your sleeve. He yearns for a relationship that feels destined, overwhelming, and irresistible. He craves mad love. So, throw caution to the wind and reveal your vulnerabilities *pronto*.

Pisces needs to see your humanness, bond with it, and be able to flow with it. Do the same back by using your intuition to read and compliment his energy. Understand his subtle forms of communication, like reading his body language correctly and responding back properly. It'll be those details that'll mesmerize him. Don't get pushy, though; he hates arrogance and aggression. Be soothing, charming, playful, and most of all, a bit self-deprecating. He's the sign of the fish, so use this as a metaphor. Work with the flow, gently luring him in with your delicious bait and then wait for him to bite.

Loving Him in the Boudoir

Pisces is a notch not to be missed, as he's got a way of melting into you that's so natural and right that it almost feels masturbatory. Gifted with amazing instincts, in bed he'll have an uncanny ability to feel your needs to do you right. Seeing that he loves to please and show off his skill to know you on an ethereal level, this talent is most gratifying for his lovers. No matter what the circumstances are though, he'll always strive to give sex as if there's something real between you, even if it's just for that moment. Sex to Pisces is another facet in deepening a connection and communicating his passion. The intensity of which he performs is a direct correlation of his emotions, as they fuel him. In fact, it'd be impossible for him to do anything or anyone he doesn't feel.

As if that weren't enough, Pisces is a sappy romantic. He's all about the flowers, wine, and poetry. He lives to get lost in a fantasy and aims to make his sexual encounters saturated with imagination, passion, and beauty—anything to make a soul drift away into a dreamy wonderland that's more than just orgasms. He understands the importance of memory and creating legacies, making him a perfectionist when it comes to marking his amorous territory. The more you matter, the more creativity he'll put into every aspect of the sex—before, after, and during. With no limits to what he'll do in the name of love, it makes him too precious for words.

MAKING HIM COME TO THE
PALM OF YOUR HAND

Eye Candy

Despite all his spiritual mumble jumble, Pisces is a guy that bows down to the power of pretty. So, pull out your finest vestments when it comes to thrilling him. He knows presentation matters; as it's your calling card to the world—and the message he's looking to receive reeks of romance, playfulness, and innocence with a tinge of flamboyance sprinkled in for good measure. If you want to adorn yourself in tasteful status symbols, go for it. He has a secret penchant for that kind of stuff too. It shows you have an indulgent side, which means the chances are high you'll spoil him too. To wrap it all into place, keep a humble attitude, as sweet arm candy is what he craves.

Stylin' Seduction:

- ♡ Soft colors. Wear off-white, pastel pink, blue, or green to grab his attention and appeal to his romantic core.
- ♡ Designer labels and valuable accessories. Look like a forlorn jet-set victim. While he isn't superficial per se, he does like to be taken care of—and no one does it better than someone who puts out the big bucks to look nice.
- ♡ Au naturel style, plain with simple colors and a flattering fit. A palette for your soul to shine from.
- ♡ Vintage. There's romance in retro.
- ♡ Plush fabrics, such as velvet or even fleece. Anything comforting to the touch.
- ♡ Playful socks and nice shoes. He's the ruler of the feet and loves anything related to them.
- ♡ Costumes or outfits with a playfulness. He likes creative dressing.

Tasty Treats

Food

Despite his what his lithe body would portray, he's a pig. His appetite is big and his tastes are decadent. Typically born with a refined tongue, Pisces is attuned to the subtlest tastes that make him a true gourmet. Understand food can transport him to other levels of consciousness, so think of restaurants like temples; the more exotic, rich, and complex the flavors they provide, the more he'll transcend into happiness. Also note, most Pisces will blow their budgets on good food. He lives well by eating well; food is his legal high.

Erotic Eats:

♡ Sushi. He's the sign of the fish.

♡ Any waterfront location that serves seafood. This could be lakefront, seaside, or somewhere by a pond or waterfall.

♡ Private rooms in fancy restaurants where it's all about being pampered.

♡ Haute couture cuisine with top chefs. He loves the finest of the finest and his palate is developed for sophistication. Indulge him; he'll be putty in your hands.

♡ Any restaurant with a good bar. He's into his fancy drinks, so any place with a good martini menu, fun daiquiris, or exclusive wine list will do fine.

♡ Foreign cuisine. He loves cultural adventures and is always game to try new foods.

♡ Dinner theater. Something imaginative and edible, what better combo could he ask for!

Movies

All Pisces want a one-way ticket to Fantasy Island. Since none of them are going to get it, going to the movies is close enough.

Spending most of his life daydreaming away, movies offer guided tours to alternate realities that are as real as life when played out on the big screen. Plus, he's a big ole sap ball and he loves to be swung through the emotional spectrum when he can. To him, emotions are like muscles that he must exercise to get the most out of them. The heavier the intensity, the better the reward.

Cinematic Foreplay:

- ♡ Super-high drama. He gets a lot out of emotional purging.
- ♡ Musical theater. He loves anything that involves dance.
- ♡ Horror and suspense. The rush thrills him.
- ♡ Erotica. Anything sensual but tasteful is his speed.
- ♡ Spiritually themed movies. He's all about expanding and raising his consciousness.
- ♡ Comedy. If he's in a bad mood, it lifts him right up.
- ♡ Fantasy or sci-fi. He lives in an alternate universe anyway and relates well to this genre.

Dating Ideas

Being that Pisces is the finale of the zodiac, he's touted as an old soul. On a good day, this can be expressed by his incredible ability to persevere despite any obstacles, complete with an optimistic attitude and a deeply loving appreciation for every moment. On a bad day, though, he'll resemble that of an old man too tired and over it. In the honeymoon phase of dating, though, you should expect only continuous good days with him and plan accordingly. To avoid his mood from tanking, activities that he'll thrive in are creative pursuits, low-impact nature exploring, decadent indulgences, or anything flamboyant and romantic.

Playful Planning:

♡ Dancing. He can't resist it. Throw in the booze and you'll be out until sunrise!

♡ Water. Anything near a body of water will bring out his romantic side. This could mean having a picnic and reading him your favorite poetry by the ocean or renting a paddle-boat and cruising a lake. After all, he's a water sign.

♡ A spa day. He loves to be pampered and won't be able to resist seeing you all oiled up.

♡ Aquatic theme adventure. Swim with dolphins, whale-watch, or visit an aquarium.

♡ Botanical gardens. The lush prettiness will intoxicate him.

♡ A spiritual retreat. A group meditation and things of that nature will be sure to please.

♡ Make art together—like painting, song, film, etc. Or even find a cool locale and get two disposable cameras and see how you both see the world.

Sound Seduction

Conversation

Upon first contact, Pisces may come off a bit shy or snotty, but once you get him rolling you'll learn he's a talker. While he can certainly hold court fabulously, he doesn't tend to want to hog the scene, as he isn't egotistically driven and will prefer conversations that are deeply personal and get to the meat of who you are. He likes hearing about what makes you tick and also sharing his innermost feelings. With Pisces, communication is for bonding, and whichever words can do it, spill them out. Show him a piece of your soul and he'll show you his.

Icebreakers:

- ♋ Discuss spiritual beliefs. He's usually rooted in some spiritual practice and will love expanding on it with you.
- ♡ Talk about art: his favorite pieces and artists. Creativity and imagination are his fuel.
- ♋ Find out what's his idea of love. What's the most romantic thing he's ever done and been done for him? He loves talking about his memories, especially if they involve romance.
- ♡ Bring up karma and ask him what he thinks his next life will be like. See how creative or cuckoo he is!
- ♡ Ask him to reveal a big turning point in his life. He usually had some type of major awakening in life. If he not, be cautious. A Pisces not on a path of evolution is a loose cannon.
- ♡ Ask him about freaky psychic experiences. Pisces have a heightened intuition and are bound to have several creepy happenings to share.
- ♡ Talk about the past. This can prove a never-ending resource of discussion: his or the world's. Ask him what historical event or period he would of liked to witness or parts of his life he'd relive.

Music

Music is like breathing for Pisces, a complete necessity. After all, how can his life unravel properly without the right soundtrack to emphasize his moods and innermost feelings? It can't and that's why he prefers constantly listening to music, as it heightens his feelings to a higher level of awareness and makes his surroundings and situation more intense. Not to say his music tastes are always heavy, because he does have a great sense of humor and loves irony. No matter, the music he'll gravitate to will be the kind that forces out feelings and create moods, by being overpowering, intense, or incredibly melodic and pretty.

Mood Makers:

- ♡ Dance and funk music. If he can dance to it, he'll love it.
- ♡ Religious chants. He's got a spiritual side to him.
- ♡ Eastern music, bhangra. Anything exotic will appeal to him.
- ♡ Cheesy pop and/or over-the-top chanteuses. Think ballads and anything full of feeling.
- ♡ Acoustic and folk. Music with confessional lyrics and somber emotions speak to him.
- ♡ Psychedelic rock, trance, or reggae. Any music that's associated with altered states.
- ♡ Bossa nova and samba. It's smooth and mellow, the type of vibe he'll thrive with.

Gifts

The Pisces symbol is two fishes going in opposite directions. This means he dwells at the extremes. In the gift-giving sense, he can be a greedy brat expecting tons of flash or a ridiculously modest sap lacking any shred of materialism. Typically, it'll be evident which proclivity your Pisces inhabits. However, each always has an ability to swing to the other side on a whim. Obviously, if your Pisces is into the finer things in life, you should note that he'll know quality when he sees it and which labels to coo over. If he's the Mother Teresa type, get as personal and creative as you can, as giving him a gift with personal meaning will be worth its weight in emotional gold.

Boxed Treats:

- ♡ Gifts with a spiritual significance. Ones that have been passed down to you from someone special are even better.
- ♡ Art supplies. He likes to express himself creatively one way or another.

♡ Dance lessons. Anything involving dance is sure to please.

♡ Any artistic creation where he played the muse.

♡ A photo album of all your loving memories.

♡ Body products and massage certificates. He can't resist being primped and preened.

♡ Stuff for his bed, as that's his favorite place to be. Sleep is his god.

Touch Me

Pisces wants to be swept off his feet, be flogged with absolute pleasure and pain, and have the passion ooze out of him. Show your emotional intensity and he'll get as hard as steel. By playing out your emotions as powerfully as possible, you'll bring out the hungriest and horniest devil in him, as he loves having sex as if he's a star of a prime-time soap opera. The more over the top, the hotter he gets. If you're angry, scream and yell. If you're sad, cry hysterically. Express your feelings and give him something to work with. He'll feed off that energy, as it propels him into your psyche. His sex can then be like a ladder that reaches deep into you to rescue you. Nothing beats a good orgasm to save the day, especially if he comes as the hero.

Obviously, the other variation is that he gets to act out and you can be his sexy Florence Nightingale. Not that there always has to be heavy or dramatic emotions that set the stage, as Pisces also has great comedic timing and can also do playful. At the core of it though, what stimulates him is the emotional exchange. So the more there is, the more he can get off.

Of course, with Pisces being a romantic at heart, don't forget to reveal your tender side when making love. He appreciates a delicate lover and to also be treated as such. All those stories you hear about people crying in bed from the sheer emotional intensity of the moment are probably in bed with Pisces—and you know, he loves it. So light those candles, throw about the rose pedals, put on the slinky outfits, turn on the love songs, and be ready to sexually express all the things you adore about him, and not just his fun, dirty, sweet, and sexy side, but also his loving and soft side, because that's where you'll find his real g-spot.

Ways to Heat Up Your Pisces:

♡ Pisces wants his lovers at his feet, because that's where his erogenous zone is. So lick his toes and massage his tootsies; then work your way on up and get lucky.

♡ Say you want to nap; it's the easiest way to get him to bed— but seriously, he might really fall asleep.

♡ Be sad. Play the victim and need him to be your hero or be his hero when he's sad and lonely.

♡ Put on the sleazy dance music and break out the cocktails. There's never a bad time for a champagne room atmosphere.

♡ Pull out all the romantic accoutrements: candles, flowers, wine, and all the things that would be deemed romantic. He's all for those traditions.

♡ Do him somewhere historical and possibly haunted. He gets off on otherworldly experiences.

♡ Do him in a body of water or near one. If not possible, put on a sounds of the ocean CD—corny, but it'll work.

Role-playing

Give Pisces any excuse to get all dolled up, possibly have his ass spanked, and he's there. Yes, he's a playful flirt and role-playing is second nature for him, as he's a natural-born actor. In the bedroom, his skills are heightened with a dramatic orgasm as his reward. As a fan of excess, be ready to go to extremes in costume and intense characters, because flexing his imagination is a form of foreplay. As for plots, stroke his creative side with themes that incorporate history, mythology, fantasy, or compassion. Then, play them out with operatic decadence and get ready to crescendo like you could have never imagined before.

Cast of Characters:

- ♡ Mortal with his higher self. This will appeal to his spiritual side.
- ♡ Renaissance or medieval characters (or actually any period piece fantasy). He's fascinated with the past.
- ♡ Protesters who have just completed a fast. Integrate food in this. He loves playing the martyr.
- ♡ Patient and doctor. Anytime he can play victim or help one is hot for him.
- ♡ Mythological creatures: Roman, Greek, etc. Make your own Poseidon adventure, as he loves mythology.
- ♡ A pirate on an island with a mysteriously beautiful inhabitant who is also a horny sex kitten. He loves fantasy situations.
- ♡ Widower and spirit of deceased spouse. Anything mystical will appeal to his senses.

Taking the Bait

It doesn't take a genius to figure out when Pisces is hooked. His toothbrush will be at your house right after consummation, he's doing things like celebrating your one-week anniversary, coming up with names for your kids, and gushing every time you look his way. This man loves, loves, loves to fall in love—and we are talking head over heels in love too. Being completely in touch with his emotions, he's fearless about sharing them, as he couldn't contain them even if he tried. When in love, he wants to shout it from the rooftops. He understands the miracle of finding someone he can connect with and share a state of bliss with, making him a grateful lover. With such enthusiasm, the world will know when he's in love.

For his lover, he'll know no bounds and his selfless nature will come out in full force. With everyone Pisces dates, he'll play helpless fawn to get them to spoil him or do his dirty work. This behavior is non-negotiable, as he lives to be cared for. The major difference if he loves you is he'll take care of you in return. If he shells out his wallet generously on a continual basis, understand you have something serious. In asserting this role, he's showing respect and aiming to establish a level of equality, which he'll only look to create with his true love. Yes, he'll strive for the highest level of maturity only for the one he loves, as he typically comes from a history of relationships where he let himself get treated as a baby or victim. In the face of love, he'll know better and act accordingly. By being on his best behavior, he's acknowledging true love and soul mates do exist, as it'll inspire him to take full responsibility of his actions.

As for the quality of the relationship, expect an "us against the world" attitude and crazy romantic scenarios to spark. His love is eternal and his devotion is strong, going to the ends of the universe for you and creating a breathlessly romantic story that can inspire great cinema. Pisces gives unconditional love, even to the point of you being able to walk all over him. Once in love he'll have absolutely no concept of pride. On one hand it can be a fantastically beautiful experience to witness, but on the other hand if he's wasting the worship on the wrong person, it can be just downright creepy.

UNAUTHORIZED: ASTRAL AUTOPSY

Recognizing Fear

Pisces are fearful of many things, but most of them aren't of the normal 3-D/planet Earth variety. His terrors deal with the beyond, the unexplainable, and worst of all, his own psyche. He's his own worst enemy, freaking himself out with conjuring up mystical uncertainties and a judgment day of some form—even if he's a diehard atheist. As the zodiac's legacy keeper, his concerns deal with the world outside the here and how. He lives for a bigger, deeper, and more spiritual existence than the everyday and if his faith gives out, so can he.

Main cause
The possibility of existential angst as a reality.

Immunizing His Fears:

- ♡ Back up his hunches. His intuition is strong and if you stand by his convictions he'll stick to them too.
- ♡ Show compassion to the less fortunate. Do volunteer work or cry for the handicapped on TV. Don't do the latter more than once, he'll be suspicious you're overacting.
- ♡ Have a high-paying job. He needs to know you can take care of him, even if he has his own money (aka "fun money").
- ♡ Have some sort of belief system that you rely on to explain this mess called life.
- ♡ Give him something of emotional value. By providing him a sentimental part of you to possess 24–7, it'll comfort him beyond words.

Infecting with Fear:

- ♡ Play against karma when he's around. For example, go overboard with road rage and tailgate, flip off people, and scream out the window.
- ♡ Wear open-toe shoes with ugly feet. He loves feet, but not if they're ugly.
- ♡ Make him watch a movie about possession or any other possible supernatural events that can happen. He loves horror, but if it hits to close to home, it can freak him out.

♡ Act nervous. His sensors will pick up the anxiety without your saying a word. Remember, he's a sponge for any emotion floating in the atmosphere.

♡ Break a superstition or tell him someplace is haunted. Perhaps slip out that the person who lived in your apartment ten years ago committed suicide in the bathroom.

Recognizing Anger

Pisces' life's work is finding inner peace and being one with his world, making him a product of his environment. If he's in a disruptive atmosphere, his tendency will be absorbing the frenzy. If he can't remove himself from the situation, eventually the anger will manifest itself outwardly and can take two routes. One is the complete meltdown with an intense and often exaggerated outpouring of emotions. The other more typical route is internalizing his rage, which then is expressed in two ways: a creative catharsis or self-destructive behavior. Hence, his up-fish and down-fish symbol.

Main cause
Being the only selfless person on Earth can be a maddening task.

Immunizing His Anger:

♡ Let him overhear you describe him as gorgeous. Vanity saves.

♡ Meditate with him every day and have a healthy stock of spiritual books to keep his nerves calm.

♡ Know powerful quotes from famous spiritual leaders and be ready to whip them out. It'll ease his mind, knowing he'll have this knowledge at arm's reach when times get rough.

♡ Respect his need for quiet time and know he's moody and it can happen at a drop of a hat.

♡ Don't skimp when it comes to adventure. You have to go all the way or he'll feel short-changed and unloved.

Infecting Him with Anger:

♡ Refuse to dance with him or not play the part of partner in a couple situation. Be into your independence.

♡ Rush him while he's shopping. It's one of the pleasures of his life, don't spoil it!

♡ Skuzz up his bathtub and/or use and grimy up his bath products. This is sacred ground you're messing with.

♡ Wake him up in the middle of the night periodically and keep him from his precious sleep. He loves it more than he'll ever love you. Keep him from it and beware.

♡ Leave crumbs in his bed—that's his altar.

Recognizing Sadness

Famous for his empathy, Pisces can often turn into an emotional basket case and feel as if he must carry the weight of the world. Sure, he feels deeply and will have a tendency to go into pity-party mode every time he hits a bump in the road. However, he also has a propensity to exploit his talent for compassion to manipulate, since playing victim is easier than getting off his ass. So, use your best judgment when gauging the depth of his despair and avoid coddling his so-called delicate sensibility.

Main cause

Being an emotional sponge makes him sad, but dwelling on it can make you his slave.

Immunizing His Sadness:

♡ Enjoy talking about pretend things and create a fantasyland where it's sunny all day. In this safe world, he can always hide and stay happy.

♡ When he starts to feel blue, take him to a good psychic.

Even if he suspects lies, any kind of hope to hold on to will put him into a better mind-set.

♡ Be a die-hard optimist and always find something good, even with the most horrific events. This attitude will help steer him clear of crashing into the emotional rocks, if he knows he can always find an uplifting answer through you.

♡ Take him out dancing often. Keep the endorphins pumping.

♡ Do volunteer work with him or join some kind of community initiative. Keep him happy by stocking up the karmic points together.

Infecting Him with Sorrow:

♡ Always want to eat at home. This boy needs to be wined and dined or he shrivels. Keep him at home and feed him the same things to speed up the process.

♡ Watch sad movies or play sad music. He'll get depressed through osmosis.

♡ Be grossed out by his feet and refuse to touch them. The rejection of part of him will go right to the core of his soul.

♡ When he goes into his martyr mode, ignore him. Tough love isn't his speed.

♡ Have no interest in his creative outlets, whether it's dance, gardening, and/or watercolor. Being blind to this part of him will make him feel invisible and sad, regardless of the fact that he isn't being creative for your benefit.

Recognizing Trust

Intuition is everything to Pisces. If he has a good vibe from you, then you're good to go. Then, depending on the circumstance you're in with him is how he'll gauge the depth of his trust. Not that he's making a judgment on your character, but how he doles out his trust will be based on how he can rely on you from situation to situation. He knows everyone has his or her own talents, and he'll rely on every one in a different way—based on what the signs tell him.

Main cause
It depends on the reception of his antennae, whether trust comes in loud and clear or totally fuzzy.

Immunizing His Trust:

- ♡ Always have a communist way of spending money, one for all and all for one.
- ♡ Don't be a mean citizen and do insensitive things like park in handicap parking spots, when you're aren't handicapped.
- ♡ Be superstitious. Believe in the beyond and live with karma on your mind.
- ♡ Treat everyone the same, from the cleaning lady to a CFO.
- ♡ Be respectful of the past/history.

Infecting His Trust:

- ♡ Don't be charitable and leave meager tips.
- ♡ Be into money and act the part of a total capitalist pig. Although he likes knowing he's with someone who has money, he doesn't want to think you're into it as a power.
- ♡ Never use your intuition to feel your way in and out of things. Always be by the book.
- ♡ Don't have a romantic view of life, love, or anything.
- ♡ Have no spiritual practice or revelations that create part of your makeup.

Recognizing Motivation

Considering his favorite activity is sleep, you can only imagine the might, passion, and excitement you need to get him going. To Pisces, sleep is more than just a necessity, but a doorway to a whole other world for him to escape in. Therefore, activities to keep him awake must be excessively stimulating for his body, mind, and soul. He won't do anything he doesn't feel and things he'll be inspired by only fall into these two categories: hedonistic paradise or martyr-like pursuits.

Main cause
If he doesn't move, he'll get bedsores.

Immunizing His Motivation:

- ♡ Set a schedule and don't allow him to work at his own pace. He operates best going with his own flow.
- ♡ Talk in realistic terms. He abhors reality and dealing with it in anyway.
- ♡ Have a bad feeling. He'll listen to negative omens.
- ♡ Create a sense of frigidness and squelch any room for creativity. Be overly formal.
- ♡ Tell him something is un-PC and he won't want to get involved with the bad vibes.

Infecting Him with Motivation:

- ♡ Make sure he's well rested before asking him anything to which you want a positive response.
- ♡ Have a good psychic intuition about something and he'll opt to go with it.
- ♡ Have him go into action for the needy.
- ♡ Play up the creative element of something and he's in.
- ♡ He's always up for festive activities, as long as he'll get back in time for bed. If there's booze and dancing, even better!

DESTINATION: DUMPSVILLE

Celestial Voodoo on You

Pisces would rather get a root canal on all his teeth than have to dump you and purposely make you feel bad. This makes him a slippery sucker in the getaway, always opting for the sleight-of-hand solutions rather than the obvious. However, despite how he initiates the breakup, the one thing he'll always aim to achieve is that he comes out the martyr. So beware of the sabotage, as that's the way he gets you.

It begins with little things, as Pisces likes to test the waters before going all out on his attack. At first he'll look for little foibles you make and make a bigger deal out of them than necessary. Then, as he picks up momentum, he'll get more dramatic and more hurt by random things that he'll declare as careless actions on your part. He'll twist situations around to make you seem callous. Things can be as absurd as you ordering the wrong dinner that reminds him of an ex or you suggesting a movie rental that reminds him of his dead dog.

In no time, he'll also get overly possessive and jealous, holding on to you tighter, therefore having it easier for you to trip up. As soon as you mess up enough times or fall into one of his traps, he'll then slam down his cards and declare the game over. This then makes him able to feel good about breaking up with you, like he's made some valiant effort to flee from your abusive nature. Of course, he'll probably create more pain than need be, but with Pisces, he loves nailing himself to the wall and being shot at with arrows. After all, pain is just too delicious to resist.

. . . And Other Signs He Hates You

There's a fine line between hate and love with Pisces, and sometimes even he won't know how to distinguish the two, making the scary fact of the matter that if he hates you, he might glom on to you even more. Being that he's so compassionate, driven by his emotions, and psychically in tune, he often misinterprets his own disdain for you as sympathy or an energy that he has to correct. Either way, this will launch him on to his "selfless" mission, with you as his project.

The awful thing is that Pisces can come across like he likes you even when he hates you. In feeling bad about disliking you, he'll be more driven to know you and want to understand you—trying to find any redeeming quality. After he makes a diagnosis, he'll then pick areas of you to work on (aka parts to change and attempt to make you more likable to him). In his inability to accept that not everyone has to get along and that he doesn't have to like everyone, he'll go on an obviously unnecessary psychodrama. He's known to mess with his mind and possibly mess with yours, in an effort to rebuild you to his liking. Even if you call him on it, realize that once he starts, he rarely stops, as that's not his style. His style is crash and burn.

If you're nutty enough to stick around for this, in time he'll get worn down by the frustration that you won't do as he says and he'll turn into a maniacal tyrant to prove his fruitless points. This can go back and forth until someone (usually you) takes the responsibility to walk way. However, with all this drama he has created, he now has a story to really grab on to, hate you for, and play himself as some sort of selfless victim. Sure, it's a longer and rather unwarranted route, but this is how he rolls and perhaps one day he can learn his feelings don't equal fact and he can maturely walk away with a simple, "It's not you, it's me."

Beating Him to the Punch

Throwing Pisces back to the sea can be a rather difficult process if you don't know what to expect. For a successful mission, you need to come fully prepared, emotionally immunizing yourself to possible drama of the very insane variety. Desperate acts can include major water works or suicide threats, as Pisces loves throwing himself upon the funeral pyre. As long as you're ready for this emotional manipulation and can protect yourself accordingly, the rest is easy.

He gets off on theatrics and pouring guilt on thick, as this is how he responds to pain. Even if Pisces pleads his endless love, ignore it. Sure, he might mean it for the moment, but typically he'll talk out of his ass when desperate. In time, he'll tire himself out and hit rock bottom with his patheticness that'll typically make him so mesmerizingly miserable that he'll use it to pull at the heartstrings of some other unsuspecting sucker to feel sorry for him and nurse his wounds.

The truth about Pisces is that he's a serial dater and doesn't like the single life (unless he's one of those ascetic Pisces who is all about suffering). So, in actuality, you're doing him a favor, giving him the fodder he needs to find a new lover who can rebuild him and be selflessly devoted to him, while he sucks up their generosity. Like his symbol of the two fish, Pisces has to go down to get back up, and this is sometimes the sick way he goes about it. Thankfully, for him, the world is full of fools who will love him.

Ridding Yourself of Pisces with Minimal Scarring:

- ♡ Be uncreative and have no room for fun.
- ♡ Spoil yourself, but be cheap with him. Pisces wants to be pampered, and in his eyes, how well you do it is a total reflection on your feelings for him and your character.
- ♡ Be a total work-a-holic and use that as your excuse, but don't apologize for it. He'll try to compete, but he knows in the end that he'll lose and won't fight.
- ♡ Show no depth of emotion and least of all, any shred of compassion. Like, laugh at all the bad things on the news.
- ♡ Tell him that his problems and demands are ridiculous. He hates feeling ridiculed for his "sensitivity."

♡ He's vain and overly sensitive. With six words you can unhook him: "I no longer find you attractive."

♡ Don't sleep in the same bed. Go home after sex and tell him you prefer sleeping alone.

Kick, Drop, and Kill

Pisces is the sign of inheritances; so, expect to be left behind with something—anything from a headache to enough karmic points to get you through fabulously for the next several lifetimes, even if you're a serial killer in all of them. The fact is, being with Pisces and not winning at the game of love isn't easy. Your patience, time, self-worth, intelligence, kindness, boundaries, finances—everything gets tested. He can be a black-hole kind of lover—invisibly and slowly sucking you dry of all your defenses. The more you're compressed, the more exaggerated your worst fears will feel, kind of like being forced into a scared-straight program for relationships.

Being that Pisces goes at it with the intensity of a kamikaze, surviving one means you have successfully been able to swim back from an infinite abyss of self-hatred, learned how to create limits, and accepted your level of compassion that's comfortable for you. In the end, you really get to understand the capability of your heart. Hell, even if you realize it's totally black, you can accept it as okay because that's who you are. Regardless of your possible heartlessness, though, the biggest gift will come in the form of understanding how sane you truly are, as you-know-who will betroth you an infallible reference point to what "crazy" will act, look, smell, sound, and feel like—and what can be more priceless than that?

ABOUT THE AUTHOR

This is Kiki's second book. Her first is *Angst:
Teen Verses from the Edge,* which she co-edited.
She lives in NYC and can be reached at
astrosexologistkiki@gmail.com.